pмs, peʀimenopause, and ʏou

PMS, Perimenopause, and YOU

A GUIDE TO THE EMOTIONAL, MENTAL, AND PHYSICAL PATTERNS OF A WOMAN'S LIFE

Updated from the previous edition,
The PMS & Perimenopause Sourcebook

LORI A. FUTTERMAN, R.N., PH.D.
JOHN E. JONES, PH.D.

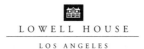

LOWELL HOUSE

LOS ANGELES

NTC/Contemporary Publishing Group

618.172
F996 p

Library of Congress Cataloging in Publication Data

Futterman, Lori A.
  PMS, perimenopause, and you : a guide to the emotional, mental, and physical patterns of a woman's life / Lori A. Futterman, John E. Jones.— 2nd ed.
    p. cm.
  Previously published as: PMS & perimenopause sourcebook.
  Includes bibliographical references and index.
  ISBN 0-7373-0511-8 (pbk.)
    1. Premenstrual syndrome—Popular works. 2. Menstruation disorders—Popular works. I. Jones, John E. II. Futterman, Lori A. PMS & perimenopause sourcebook. III. Title.

RG165.F88 2000
618.1'72—dc21   00-057934

Design by Laurie Young

Published by Lowell House
A division of NTC/Contemporary Publishing Group, Inc.
4255 West Touhy Avenue, Lincolnwood, Illinois 60712, U.S.A.

Printed in the United States of America

International Standard Book Number: 0-7373-0511-8
00 01 02 03 04 DHD 18 17 16 15 14 13 12 11 10 9 8 7 6 5 4 3 2 1

contents

foreword

Premenstrual syndrome (PMS) has remained an enigma, despite a plethora of theories and increasing clinical and research attention. In 1980, I was co-convenor of a meeting of international experts on PMS held in Berlin, Germany, at the time of a congress of the International Society of Psychosomatic Obstetrics and Gynecology. Each expert presented a summation of his or her research findings. However, during the open discussion session, each was asked for a definition of PMS, and each presented a different definition. Little wonder that there was such discrepancy in their findings and recommendations.

Twenty years later, we still have a discrepancy in terms ranging from PMS, to premenstrual tension (PMT), to premenstrual dysphoric disorder (PMDD). Some of us have even loosely used the abbreviation PMS to read "premenopausal syndrome." The term *syndrome* usually represents a group of symptoms with a common cause. In this instance, the confusion in the medical literature, which consequently translates into confusion for women, most likely is due to the fact that there is not one, but several potential disorders.

Lori Futterman and John Jones have succeeded remarkably well in translating the medical literature into a coherent and valuable resource for women. They have, moreover, utilized their clinical experience well, with a series of real-life patient examples. Their real achievement in this book is twofold: They provide a lucent explanation of normal physiology, that is, the exquisite interaction between the various mechanisms that ensure our normal mind and body function; and they demonstrate how these mechanisms can sometimes move out of synchrony and, even in the absence of any organic disease, still trigger altered mind or body responses. In this way, they demonstrate that a syndrome such as PMS can occur in even the "healthiest" individual.

Understanding a phenomenon leads to the next logical step: learning to deal with it. Unfortunately, accepting and dealing with a situation does not necessarily mean that a cure is always possible, but at least the situation can be understood and perhaps tolerated.

In *PMS, Perimenopause, and You*, the potential effects of various treatments are placed in perspective. These treatments are broad in range, vary in effectiveness, and often work together to enhance each other's effect. A clear message in this book is the value of a holistic approach and healthy living.

Despite rapid advances in technology, biomedicine, drug development, and potentially gene therapy, we should never forget that for every potential disease or bodily change there may be an emotional response. The way we react to any physiological or pathological alteration is therefore affected by social, cultural, and psychological factors. The sum of the hormonal and psychosocial cultural factors then becomes the "clinical syndrome." Clinical management thus requires recognition of all these factors, and clearly physical and emotional components must receive equal doses of attention if a successful outcome is to be achieved. *PMS, Perimenopause, and You* succeeds admirably in explaining these interactions and providing mechanisms for dealing with them. In over thirty years of clinical practice, one observation stands foremost in my mind: that an informed patient is more likely to be motivated toward a cure and to achieve that goal. This book will help readers succeed in the first step: obtaining the required information.

Wulf H. Utian, M.D., B.Ch., Ph.D., F.R.C.O.G., F.A.C.O.G., F.I.C.S., The Arthur B. Hill Professor Emeritus, Case Western Reserve University, Cleveland, Ohio
Executive Director, The North American Menopause Society

preface

This book is intended to benefit women who are interested in understanding and managing their PMS and perimenopausal experiences. We are grateful to the many women who have shared their stories and lives with us. Their courage and openness gave us the inspiration and motivation to undertake the work.

Grateful acknowledgment is given to a number of important people who improved this book through helpful suggestions. These include Nancy Cetel, M.D.; Lori B. Futterman, B.S., B.A.; Danny Keiller, M.D.; L.C. Miccio-Fonseca, Ph.D.; Maura Laverty, R.N., M.H.S.; M. E. (Ted) Quigley, M.D.; Susan Trompeter, M.D.; and James Williams, O.M.D., L.Ac. The opinions in the book are those of the authors, and these friends should not be held accountable for any factual errors or opinions with which they or others may disagree. We heartily thank each of them for their invaluable contributions.

Lori A. Futterman, R.N., Ph.D.
John E. Jones, Ph.D.
San Diego, California

Introduction

Reflect for a few moments about your personal thoughts about what it means to be a healthy woman. Ask yourself the following questions:

What does it take to maintain personal health?

What can make you healthy or unhealthy?

How does your idea of health relate to disease?

How does health relate to the menstrual cycle?

How can you tell how healthy you are?

What about your mental health?

How do you see the connection between your mind and your body?

Now step back a bit and think about how you attempt to remain healthy. Here are some additional questions to ask yourself:

What do I do to ensure that I remain healthy?

What do I do that I know is probably unhealthy for me?

Just how healthy am I right now?

How much difficulty am I having premenstrually these days?

What body changes am I going through these days?

What symptoms am I experiencing that are related to my menstrual cycle?

What do I need to do about my health right now?

Thinking through such questions can lead you to a realization that your health is your business, that everything happening within and around you can affect your well-being. It is important for you to learn how to notice the obvious and subtle changes you experience. Monitoring yourself is your job, and you need to make sure that your health-care team takes information about you seriously as they work to fashion treatments that may help alleviate any discomfort you may be having. Family members and others may discount your concerns as well, so you need to become assertive when communicating with significant people in your life to help them understand what you may be going through. Gaining knowledge about premenstrual syndrome (PMS) and perimenopause can help you feel confident as you encounter change.

Women are conditioned to believe that if they complain about subtle bodily changes, they will be labeled as neurotic, crazy, or difficult. Problems related to your menstrual cycle, such as PMS or perimenopause, are known to affect some women's functioning so adversely that their work, home life, and relationships suffer, as well as their overall health. Maintaining balance and a sense of personal stability requires you to become an advocate for your own welfare. Your body and mind are yours to maintain, and you have a right to have others treat them with sensitivity, but making that happen is up to you.

AN ORGANIZED VIEW OF HEALTH

Consider the case of Maria. She is thirty-eight-years old, married, with a six-year-old daughter. She is an administrative assistant to one of the vice presidents of a high-tech manufacturing organization. She has a history of chronic fatigue, which she has had for several years. She is often very low in energy and feels tired and somewhat depressed most of the time. Her marriage has been conflictual lately. Her husband has become impatient with her inability to pull herself out of her funk. Her daughter is beginning to have trouble at school and frequently asks Maria, "What's wrong with you, Mommy? You don't play with me like you used to." Maria has been increasing her intake of alcohol. She tends to be receptive to the latest fad diet. Her menstrual cycles are regular, but her premenstrual symptoms have become more problematic. Her moods and energy level worsen, and she withdraws "into a shell." This change is beginning to affect her work, and her boss has asked her twice to take some time off for herself. When asked, Maria blames all of her troubles on chronic fatigue and PMS. She sees the situation as a physical problem, and she is frustrated at not being able to find a medical solution.

Maria is like a lot of women who think that PMS and perimenopause are completely physical phenomena and who seek a magic potion that will make the troubles go away. They seem unaware of the interplay between their physical and psychological symptoms and treat only half of the problem. Many women know little about the changes that occur as their ovaries age, and they appear not to link their physiological condition with their emotional state at any given moment. Maria is almost maximally stressed, and she turns to drinking and eating in an attempt to "feel better." She is rapidly approaching burnout, and the depletion of her personal energy is causing her chronic fatigue to worsen. She has a decreasing amount of energy to expend on improving herself. She is in a self-defeating cycle. Until she accepts her condition holistically, she is likely to remain in this downslide.

Many people think of health as the absence of physical disease. This myopic view fails to take into account one's well-being and mental health. Physicians have long promoted a medical model of health that emphasizes illness, medication, and surgery. More holistic views treat health in terms of physical, mental, social, and spiritual well-being. It is important to broaden your view of health to include not only what is happening within your body but also in your psychological condition and your entire life situation.

Women's bodies operate differently than men's. Various diseases are unique to women, and the fact that you have menstrual cycles and corresponding hormonal ovarian fluctuations significantly affects your overall health. The interaction between your mind and your body can determine the quality of your life. Though it may never be clear whether our life experiences are primarily determined by our genetic "wiring" or the events and relationships that we face as we pass through our life stages, it is clear that biological makeup affects personal psychology and vice versa.

Every part of your body interacts with the ebb and flow of your menstrual cycle changes. These changes occur in all internal bodily systems, such as the nervous system, the endocrine system, and the reproductive system. Other parts of your body that are affected by hormonal change include your immune, metabolic, circulatory, musculoskeletal, urinary, and respiratory systems. In turn, changes in these systems affect brain chemistry as the mind and body interact in countless ways. They influence each other inseparably. Thinking about one's self is probably best done in terms of interconnected *systems.*

Your ovaries are not the center of your being, but they significantly affect almost everything you do. They influence your mood, ways of thinking, sexual functioning, energy level, sleep patterns, appetite, and, ultimately, how you view yourself. The expression of your personality inevitably changes as your ovarian hormones fluctuate, as they do in a normal menstrual cycle or as they do more unpredictably during perimenopause. Your sense of your own "femaleness" is largely dependent on the status of your ovarian hormones at any given stage of your development. From your development as a fetus throughout your life, ovarian hormones determine much of what you will experience physically and anatomically. As a fetus, exposure to your mother's hormones begins a process of shaping your gender, which in turn leads to the development of your identity as a female. An unfolding process occurs as you age chronologically, and this process has roots in your biological makeup. This process interacts with your emerging sense of who you are to create your self-concept. In short, you are not your ovaries, but they do play a significant role in the quality of your life.

The challenge is to work through the myriad changes in your body as you age so that you maintain a satisfying level of general health and well-being. This means examining external, environmental factors that can play a part in shaping your thoughts, feelings, perceptions, and realities. Studying your entire lifestyle—exercise, nutrition, relationships, nurturance of self, work, etc.—can lead to making more informed choices about how you take personal responsibility for maintaining your health.

A Model of Physical and Mental Health

Figure 1-1 shows the major influences in your mental and physical health. You can see from this diagram that your overall health is a mixture of mental and physical health. Each of these components is in turn influenced by aspects of your body, self, and environment that are linked to each other.

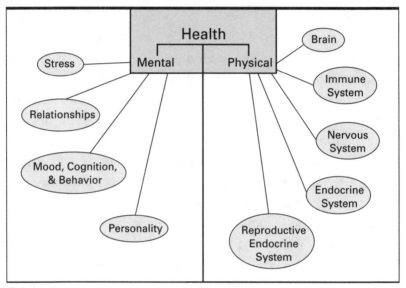

Figure 1-1

Your physical health directly involves your brain, nervous system, endocrine system (adrenal and thyroid glands), immune system, and reproductive endocrine system (ovaries). Your mental health primarily evolves from your personality (both genetic and "learned"); your moods, thinking patterns, and behavior; the quality of your relationships with others; and how you respond to internal and external conditions and events that place stress on you. The nine influencers shown in Figure 1-1 are not independent, that is, they affect each other. Your physical and mental health are, in a sense, inseparable.

On the physical side, you have five elements that interact.

1. Your brain—particularly, its chemistry—determines in large part how you think and behave. It also directs your mood states.

2. In addition, it is chemically bonded to your ovaries and adrenal and thyroid glands, thus affecting your hormonal condition.

3. Your immune system responds to environmental stress, and it protects your body against disease. If you experience prolonged stress, your thymus gland can be affected negatively, and this in turn can adversely affect your adrenal gland, the source of some of your important hormones.

4. Your nervous system regulates the brain and connects your internal systems to the external environment. Your eyesight, for example, flows through your optic nerve to the brain, where the image is rapidly and unconsciously interpreted. Much of your menstrual-related symptoms involve your nervous system as well as your mental interpretation of events.

5. Your reproductive capability is directly related to the status of your ovaries. Your physical health, then, is a function of how well your brain, endocrine, immune, nervous, and reproductive endocrine systems work together, in addition to the condition of your cardio-vascular, respiratory, musculoskeletal, urinary, and metabolic systems.

On the mental side are four elements that not only interact with each other but also with all the physical ones. Your personality includes:

1. Your sense of self
2. Your predictable patterns of behavior
3. Your way of looking at the world
4. The sum total of your life experiences

It represents your unique integration of what is privately yours—your values, philosophy, perceptions, prejudices, habits, religious outlook, likes and dislikes, among other things. Where you are on your life journey can be viewed partly as a result of the expression of your personality. As you progress through life stages the emotional challenges change, and your personality gets "lived out" through your responses to these events. Your moods and cognitions (thinking patterns) are a dramatic example of how your mental and physical processes are inseparably intertwined. The links between mood, brain chemistry, hormones, personality, and behavior are clearly established. A complicating factor in many women's lives is relationships with others, particularly partners and other family members. Friends and coworkers can also affect one's mental health, for better or worse. It is important to develop the ability to talk with people who are significant to you in order to solicit their understanding and support as you go through the aging process and to maintain your mental vitality by keeping such relationships "clean." Stress seriously affects your mental health. Excessive stress can, of course, lead to physical illness, so learning how to cope with it effectively will improve both your mental and physical health.

The health model, then, says that your overall health involves these nine elements that you need to take responsibility for. The fact that you are going through cyclical hormonal fluctuations means that you are in a constantly changing hormonal environment that affects all of your internal systems and is affected by forces in your external environment. That can make achieving complete health difficult. The interconnectedness among these systems causes your adjustments to be sometimes problematical. You may need to consult with both physicians and psychological professionals as you take charge of developing the ability to maintain your overall well-being holistically. Since these elements interact with each other, it is equally important to monitor how you are doing on each as you work through the many changes that face you as your ovaries age.

Research has shown that numerous factors affect health. Among them are genetic makeup, nutrition, exercise, stress, response to the social environment, attitudes and beliefs, emotions, and physiological change. If health means being "in synch," then it is important to learn how to read the signals that might predict imbalance and take appropriate preventive action. In this book we will specify the bodily and emotional cues that you can use to take action to maintain equilibrium. If you notice that you are being unusually irritable, for example, or you wake up with a night sweat, you may decide to monitor the symptom and seek assistance if it persists. Ovarian change can cause significant effects in your whole life situation, causing you to enter a state of imbalance, although such change may be "normal." When your ovarian and adrenal hormones fluctuate, you automatically respond, and it is important to know how these processes work so that you can make adjustments accordingly. Staying healthy, then, means maintaining awareness of both subtle and obvious changes within and around you and taking personal responsibility to do the things necessary to synchronize your activities, physical condition, and psychological state.

CHANGE IS TO BE EXPECTED

Two women are discussing their problems with premenstrual symptoms. Sally is about thirty, and Jean is about forty-five. They work together and are on their lunch break. Their eating area is somewhat private, so they talk freely with each other.

Sally: "For the past few days I have been a real grump, and I'm having a lot of trouble concentrating on my work. I have been craving sweets like crazy. I think I'm about to get my period."

Jean: "I get irritable, too, before that time. Lately I've been noticing that I am forgetting things, not remembering people's names or things I'm supposed to do. It happens a lot. My periods are totally unpredictable."

Sally: "Mine are regular, but I am noticing that my symptoms are happening for about ten days out of the month. It used to be just for five days."

Jean: "Just wait until you have periods like mine. The flow is so heavy at some times, and other times I think it'll never come."

Sally: "So how do you plan anything?"

Jean: "I can't. That's just it. On our last vacation I spent three days dealing with heavy flow. I had hoped that the trip would be romantic, but we couldn't even count on hiking or swimming for more than a few minutes."

Sally: "That must have been a real drag. I'm sure you were really disappointed. The main change that I have been noticing, besides my moods, is that I have trouble falling asleep and staying asleep through the night just before I get my period."

Jean: "I have that more days than not. Sometimes I wake up with hot sweats. It seems like the symptoms I used to experience before my periods are more intense now."

Sally: "I don't look forward to that. If my symptoms get any worse, my family might disown me."

Jean: "I'm trying to understand what's happening to me so that I can explain it to the people around me, but I am so preoccupied with coping with it, I haven't figured it out yet."

This brief exchange illustrates that women can expect changes in their premenstrual experience throughout a lifetime of menstrual cycles. The ovaries change, and corresponding changes occur in almost all aspects of your life situation. The quality of your life is dependent on the interaction between these physiological changes and the corresponding shifts that you experience in your personal psychology.

Stability in the world you create is an illusion. The only constant is change. This reality creates a situation in which you must commit to a lifelong journey of adjusting and choosing. You have to achieve a sense of balance and constancy while you experience sensual, social, emotional, and physiological changes. Today's life stressors are magnified, since the pace of living has speeded up for many people. You may become caught in the "superwoman" situation, in which you attempt to juggle work, home, recreation, exercise, and maintenance of yourself while others place conflicting demands upon you. You can expect to go through developmental stages that have never been traveled before. Stability, then, is wholly within yourself. You alone are responsible for generating a solid core of personal strength that can carry you through changes that no one can predict.

Your ovaries change continually from the time you are conceived through the time when you no longer have periods. This can be termed your ovaries' "life span." During this time your ovaries release varying levels of hormones. Those variations show up in the form of diverse symptoms, so you can expect alterations both in the types of PMS symptoms and the degree of discomfort.

The one constant throughout the life span of your ovaries is change. Not only does your body change, but you also change emotionally, socially, intellectually, and in many other ways. Change can be fluid (you flow with it) or stagnating (it takes your energy). You can embrace change, resist it, or learn how to adapt to it. How you respond to change in your life is an important part of your effectiveness as a person. Since you can count on your body changing as you age, you have the opportunity to grow psychologically at the same time. The Chinese characters for change are "danger" and "opportunity." Change, then, simultaneously represents something risky and challenging. By accepting the fact that you will have symptoms related to changes in your menstrual cycle, you can develop a better ability to work with the changes rather than be driven by them.

Today's life expectancy is over seventy years and rising. Tremendous breakthroughs in medicine are responsible for the rise in overall health of our society. Immunizations, antibiotics, innovations in the treatment of diabetes, surgical interventions such as organ transplants, and advances in the treatment of heart disease have extended the lives of countless people. However, subtle conditions that may arise because of hormonal changes have not received the same level of attention. These include pain-related conditions, osteoporosis, migraine headaches, vaginal/urinary/ bladder conditions, chronic fatigue, and others.

Health, then, is not only a state of being but also a way of living. The goal of remaining healthy requires preventing illness, strengthening your immunity to sickness, and nurturing your sense of self. This involves paying close attention to your nutrition, exercise, relationships, hormone-related symptoms, and career. You are healthy if you are able to do the things you want to, have a strong sense of inner calm, and are able to face unforeseen events that may be stressful with resolve and resourcefulness. You may achieve inner peace through meditation, religion, reflection, study of philosophy, or visualization. Having a sense of internal quiet can give you a sense of safety and can be a source of strength in coping with change. Being healthy means having uncluttered energy available to you. You are able to "rise to the occasion," and you can also choose not to engage in de-energizing behaviors such as arguments, feeling sorry for yourself, or nonproductive habits.

IS IT ALL IN YOUR HEAD?

Look at the following list and ask yourself which of these statements is true for you from time to time. These are actual complaints from women who are experiencing either premenstrual or perimenopausal symptoms.

I rant and rave.

I get hysterical, and I can't stop it.

I'm not sleeping well.

I wake up hot and sweaty.

I forget people's names.

I lost my way driving.

I don't want to be touched.

I don't have the sexual desire I used to.

I take things personally, when perhaps I shouldn't, and I overreact.

I can't concentrate.

My "get up and go" is missing.

I get tearful at funny movies.

I want sex, but don't touch me.

I feel tense and jittery a lot of the time.

I feel like I could jump out of my skin.

My sleep pattern is all out of kilter.

Sometimes I'd do anything for chocolate.

I just crave junk food.

When I feel bloated, it's almost like I'm coming out of my clothes.

I cry at the drop of a hat.

Notice that this list, although not exhaustive, includes both physical and emotional symptoms. Both PMS and perimenopause come in response to physical alterations that occur in relation to your menstrual cycle and your emotional reactions to these changes. Your personality, stress, culture, and relationships influence them. The myth that PMS and perimenopause are "all in your head" implies that they both are completely psychologically based. Such complaints as the ones in this list come from real, not imagined, sources. In other words, it's *not* all in your head.

YOUR BRAIN, NERVOUS SYSTEM, AND OVARIES

Think of your brain as your control center. It contains all your memories, your impulses, your self-protective mechanisms, and your ways of perceiving the world and attributing meaning to it. The brain calls up your emotions, such as laughing, crying, and feeling good. The parts of the brain interact continuously with one another and with all of the systems of your body. Your brain governs everything you do, feel, and think, including those things that are below the level of consciousness.

The brain gets its information through the nervous system, in the form of chemical messages. Our senses send information in, and the brain interprets these signals extremely rapidly. As a result you are mobilized to defend yourself at any moment, you may experience a mood change, or you may not even be aware that you are reacting to your environment and your brain's interpretation of it. In addition, the brain monitors systems within the body and attempts to regulate them in order to maintain health.

The brain has many communication centers that send out electrical impulses that cause the release of chemical substances. These provide information to body cells and tissues, which "talk back" to the brain. The biochemical substances that facilitate this communication are classified as neurotransmitters, neuropeptides, hormones, growth factors, and lymphokines. We will concentrate on neurotransmitters and hormones and the effects that they can have on your premenstrual and perimenopausal symptoms. Your brain, nervous system, and reproductive system, then, interact continuously.

The part of the brain that has the closest communication with your ovaries is the hypothalamus. This is governed by your pituitary gland, which responds to the rhythms of your ovaries and signals your brain to regulate the ovarian hormones, including estrogen, progesterone, and testosterone. This pituitary-hypothalamic-ovarian interaction governs the amount of hormones released into your bloodstream. This interaction is a key example of how the mind and body relate to each other on intricate levels. The interaction is affected by a number of environmental factors, including stress, diet, socioeconomic status, emotional makeup, and physiological makeup. In Chapter 2 we will detail how the levels of the three ovarian hormones relate to your experience of PMS and perimenopause. We will also discuss the effects of stress and life events affecting ovarian change in Chapter 6.

This book shows you how to pay attention to the subtle changes that you are likely to experience as your ovaries age and as you respond to change in your life situation. We will explore both your mental and physical health as we consider the facts about your unique physiology and how change can affect almost every aspect of your life.

Both PMS (the premenstrual syndrome) and perimenopause (the changes you encounter as you approach the cessation of menses) have been studied extensively, and we will review the available evidence on them. We will add observations from our extensive clinical experience in working with women who are having difficulty with these two conditions.

HOW THIS BOOK IS ORGANIZED

This book takes the approach that your experience of premenstrual and perimenopausal symptoms is best thought of holistically. That is, we will consider all aspects of your well-being, including physical, emotional, social, and spiritual. Both PMS and perimenopause are naturally occurring ovarian-related experiences. Both can, however, cause significant disruption in your life.

We will include numerous suggestions to help manage these life experiences effectively.

Chapter 1 outlines our basic approach to how the mind and body interact and how both relate to your experience of PMS and perimenopause. Chapter 2 looks at the life cycle of your ovaries, and Chapter 3 explores how your ovarian hormones are connected to such emotional states as depression and anxiety. In Chapter 4 we turn to a concern that many women have from time to time: Am I Losing My Mind?

Chapter 5 examines the notion of living through a continuum. We then turn to the connection between ovarian change and stressful life events in Chapter 6. In Chapter 7 we will review our research on PMS severity, and Chapter 8 lays out the essential features of perimenopause, or the transition into menopause.

Chapter 9 discusses relationships and how they can be affected by PMS and perimenopause; while Chapter 10 turns to the interactions of hysterectomy, oopherectomy, PMS, and perimenopause. Chapter 11 explores how PMS and perimenopause can influence sexual functioning and satisfaction. In Chapter 12 we will look at the beauty of aging. Finally, we will conclude in Chapter 13 with suggestions for managing PMS and perimenopause. The goal of this book is to give you solid, current, understandable information and encourage you to take charge of those aspects of life you can control in order to have a high quality of life in the midst of change.

WHY WE WROTE THIS BOOK

Women of all ages need to be educated regarding how their bodies change as they age and what happens to them as they live through premenstrual discomfort. We have been conducting research on women and their menstrual cycles for a number of years, and we wanted to share what we have found in a form that provides women with information they can use on a daily basis. We see ovarian change on a continuum, and part of our motivation for writing this book was to explain this way of thinking about how women's menstrual cycles and symptoms change as their ovaries age. Perimenopause has not been treated as a recognizable life stage that women pass through, and we wanted to give it the attention it deserves. Dr. Futterman sees women in psychotherapy who suffer significant distress from PMS and perimenopausal symptoms. She has observed hundreds of women as they learned how to take charge of their mental and physical health. She wanted to pass along to other women what she has learned from her clinical practice over the past thirteen years.

The intent behind this book is to provide useful information and a sense of hope to women who experience discomfort and concern about their menstrual cycles. We strongly believe that there are many proactive steps that women can take to improve their emotions, thinking, physical symptoms, and overall well-being. Women have shared stories about how PMS and perimenopausal symptoms have affected their lives, and we believe that their lifestyles have affected their symptoms as well. Women need to take personal responsibility for staying informed about their changing physiology and their options for treatment of PMS and perimenopause difficulties. If this book contributes to that end, we are glad that we took the time to research and write what is known about these two challenging conditions.

Your changing
ovaries

Think for a few moments about your development as a woman. Since the time before you were born, your ovaries have been undergoing changes that you may not have always been aware of. Here are some questions to help you access some ovarian-related incidents and developments in your life up to this point:

As a young girl, when did you first notice that you were decidedly different from boys?

When did you begin to develop breasts?

When did body hair begin to appear?

When did you notice your first vaginal discharge?

What was it like getting your first period?

How frequent were your first periods?

How did your menstrual cycle change during adolescence and early adulthood?

What premenstrual symptoms have you experienced?

If you are older, how have these symptoms changed?

How predictable are your menses these days?

Have you experienced changes in menstrual flow?

What new symptoms have emerged as you approach menopause?

Reflecting upon these questions may make you conscious that many of the changes you have experienced during your life are related to your ovarian condition. In this chapter we will explore how your ovaries function, what they produce, and how they change with age. Ovaries have a life span of their own, beginning prenatally and maturing as you age. We will describe the phases of your cycle, how the levels of ovarian hormones shift during your cycle, the ways in which your cycle changes up to menopause, and how all this is reflected in symptoms that are associated with PMS and perimenopause.

A BRIEF ANATOMY REVIEW

Figure 2-1 illustrates the parts of the body that we will focus on in the coming chapters. These are the structures that largely make up your "femaleness." Your uterus is directly tied to your ovaries, where your ova (eggs) reside, by the fallopian tubes. The endometrium, which is sloughed off as your period begins, lines the inside of the uterus. Your cervix is at the top of your vagina, and your urethra is attached to the opening of the vagina.

The ovaries are the focus of this chapter, since their welfare affects your premenstrual and perimenopausal symptoms.

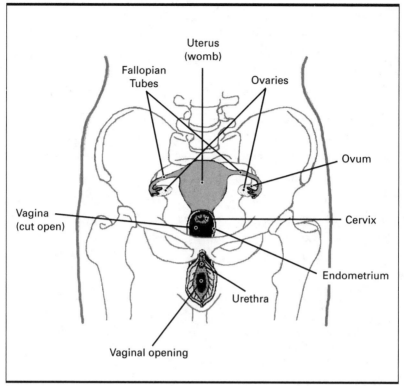

Figure 2-1

YOUR MENSTRUAL CYCLE

For many women, menstruation governs much of their daily life and planning. From the time of your first period, you anticipate the next one. As an older child or adolescent, you may have compared yourself to your friends in terms of whether you began earlier or later. Menstruation became an important part of being female, with significant symbolic meaning. Getting your period may have become inseparably intertwined with your attitudes about self, sexuality, and reproduction. You may have learned to work around your period, planning activities accordingly. You became accustomed to an emerging cycle with its ebb and flow of physical and psychological effects. Women who have been hysterectomized, with ovaries intact, often need to learn how to adjust to a "new rhythm." Even though they no longer have periods, they still have recognizable hormonal fluctuations.

Most women who have normal menstruation have a somewhat predictable cycle. Of course, some women have undergone what is referred to as surgically induced menopause (removal of the ovaries, or oophorectomy), and they do not have menstrual cycles. A very small number of women are born without ovaries or have nonfunctional ones and do not have menstrual cycles either. But if you menstruate, you have a cycle, and there are four phases that you go through each month, which averages twenty-eight days long (the "lunar month").

PHASE OF CYCLE	FOLLICULAR	OVULATORY	LUTEAL	MENSTRUAL
Average Number of Days	12–13	2	8–11	3–5

Table 2-1

Follicular Phase. The hypothalamus-pituitary complex generates a hormone called *follicle stimulating hormone* (FSH). This substance stimulates cells within the ovaries, called follicles, to produce estrogen. Once the estrogen level has risen to a sufficient amount, all but one of these follicles shrink, leaving the remaining one to become an egg.

Ovulatory Phase. This surviving follicle enlarges and ruptures under the stimulation of the pituitary's luteinizing hormone (LH). This hormone also stimulates the production of testosterone,

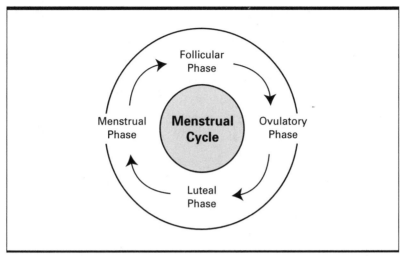

Figure 2-2

which peaks during this phase. The egg then develops into the corpus luteum, which releases progesterone. During this phase, the egg breaks loose to enter the fallopian tube, which can cause a feeling of pain termed *mittelschmerz.*

Luteal Phase. This phase is dominated by another hormone produced by the ovaries—progesterone. When the progesterone level peaks, estrogen rises again from its low level during the ovulatory phase. Both then begin to decline. Progesterone helps the body to sustain and nourish pregnancy. During this phase, testosterone probably decreases as well. By this time, your body has prepared itself for pregnancy. If the egg is not fertilized, the corpus luteum begins to break apart.

Menstrual Phase. The rapid loss of progesterone triggers the bleeding that signals the beginning of the menstrual phase. Both progesterone and estrogen reach their lowest points during this phase.

Table 2-2 summarizes the changes in ovarian hormones during a normal menstrual cycle. In the chart the terms "low" and "high" are relative terms; they vary from woman to woman. The chart illustrates how these hormones vary in relation to each other within the phases of the cycle. Estrogen and progesterone are the dominant ovarian hormones, and testosterone is considered secondary.

	PHASE OF YOUR CYCLE	FOLLICULAR	OVULATORY	LUTEAL	MENSTRUAL
HORMONE	**Estrogen**	Rises to high level	Peaks	Declines, rises again to a level below that of the follicular phase	Drops to low point, then begins to increase
	Progesterone	Low	Begins to increase	Peaks, higher than estrogen	Drops to low point, triggering menses
	Testosterone	Low	Peaks	Low, dampened by progesterone	Low

Table 2-2

DEVELOPMENTAL PHASES OF THE OVARY

The number of follicles in your ovaries declines from birth, when the average woman has about a half million. By her mid-thirties, a woman has between five and ten thousand. Since the follicles produce estrogen, this decline causes the brain to send signals to the ovaries to produce more. Eventually, when the ovaries no longer respond to increasingly higher amounts of FSH, a woman's reproductive stage typically ends at the time of menopause.

From about the age of twenty, the menstrual interval (number of days between the beginning of your periods) gradually shortens and becomes increasingly regular until you reach the perimenopausal years, or about the mid-forties. This is related to the shortening of the follicular phase of your menstrual cycle. A gradual decrease in the time between menstrual cycles occurs at about age twenty-six, with noticeable shortening around ages thirty-one to thirty-five, with the shortest cycles at three to nine years before menopause. At this time, women usually experience menstrual irregularities, which are characteristic of the transitional period known as perimenopause. Irregular bleeding, however, may be due to organic causes as well as hormonal changes and should be investigated medically. The reproductive potential of the ovary is compromised a decade or more before the complete cessation of menstruation (menopause).

There are six developmental stages within the life span of the ovary. These are fetal, prepubescent, pubescent, adolescent, young adult, midlife, and mature.

The *fetal* stage is marked by the appearance of the ovaries, along with your maximum number of follicles. There is no production of ovarian hormones, however. Gender differentiation occurs during this stage. In a sense, you have all of the "eggs" that you will ever have—before you are born. Your total number has been estimated at 400,000, of which only one-tenth of 1 percent will be used during the ovulatory process. The fetus either develops ovaries or testes, which have similar functions in that they define femaleness or maleness. The foundation for psychosexual development emerges during this stage. Genetic predispositions for various psychological conditions are put into place during the fetal stage.

During the *prepubescent* stage, the ovaries begin to release estrogen, particularly estradiol. Childhood is a quiet time for the ovaries. They develop slowly, and the effects of their development are not apparent. There is some "pre-budding" of the breasts, and there is slow maturation of the vaginal apparatus. During this stage body hair starts to develop. There may be the beginning of vaginal discharge, a yellow or white liquid that signals that menarche is on its way, probably within a year. During this stage girls learn what it means in their culture to be female, triggered by the emergence of androgens. Their genetic "wiring" becomes manifest during their early years. The combination of sex-role learning and genetic makeup is expressed in the child's unique orientation to her gender.

By age eleven to twelve, the *pubescent* stage, the production of the three ovarian hormones causes the development of secondary sex characteristics (e.g., development of breasts and pubic and underarm hair), changes in cognition, and mood shifts. With the onset of menses, premenstrual symptoms begin to appear. Puberty can begin early or late; the age span is often estimated between nine and sixteen. Menarche, or the first menstrual period, is a significant maturational event, met with either fear or joy. Young women during this stage get a "fat spurt" and gain weight. Their body composition changes, and they begin to experience body odor, which is related to the secretion of androgens by the adrenal glands. They experience a growth spurt, usually before they get their first period. Growth slows down rapidly after menarche, and their ultimate stature has been largely achieved by that time. Bone maturation and development of increased fat occur under the influence of estrogen from the ovaries.

During the *adolescent* stage, a female experiences the development of a menstrual rhythm, with more awareness of premenstrual symptoms. The adolescent cycle is erratic and characterized by longer intervals between menses. The ovulatory phase of the menstrual cycle may also be erratic, so time of ovulation is less predictable than it is later. The ovarian hormones surge during this time, and for most females this can contribute to the budding of sexual desire and arousal. The young woman's sexual organs continue to mature. Her hormonal development contributes directly to her cognitive and psychosocial development during this stage. She works out her sense of individuality as she approaches womanhood, and she must usually engage in a consideration of her moral development during this time as well.

The cycle gradually stabilizes in the *young adult* stage. The average length is twenty-eight days, but it can vary significantly among young women. For the average woman, fertility peaks during her mid-twenties. It is during this stage that the young woman's pattern of premenstrual symptoms becomes more predictable because her menses become more regular. This period is usually the peak childbearing years, and women who choose to give birth during this stage experience the significant hormonal changes associated with pregnancy.

During the *midlife* stage, roughly mid-thirties through the fourth decade, ovarian instability gradually emerges. The average length of the menstrual cycle reduces to about twenty-six days and increases in irregularity. There is a sharp drop in fertility during this stage and PMS intensifies. Perimenopause begins during the latter part of this stage, usually during the fourth decade. Menstrual flow can either become heavier or lighter at this time. Hormone levels fluctuate and decline, and cycles often become increasingly erratic. Ovulation becomes less predictable.

The *mature* stage begins with the end of the last menstrual period, or menopause. The production of the three ovarian hormones (and other hormones that the ovaries produce) reduces significantly, often to about half to two-thirds of their premenopausal levels. The ovaries slowly atrophy, and their production of important hormones gradually diminishes to insignificant amounts. This development may require hormone replacement therapy because of the dangers of osteoporosis, heart disease, and because of changes in mood, cognition, sexual functioning, and energy level.

THE OVARIAN HORMONES

Three main hormones—estrogen, progesterone, and testosterone—are produced by your ovaries, along with small amounts of other hormones. The main hormones affect your mood, energy level, thought processes, sexual desires and behavior, eating behavior, and quality of sleep. They also induce various physical symptoms, such as cardiovascular changes (palpitations, vasomotor instability, hot flushes), joint aches and pains, bone and mineral-content loss, decrease in muscle strength, and immune system deficiencies. Having improper levels of the three main ovarian hormones can increase the intensity of your premenstrual and perimenopausal symptoms. Each ovarian hormone has a corresponding receptor area in the brain and can affect the production of neurotransmitters that regulate mood and behavior.

These hormones have an effect on other mood-altering substances, called neuropeptides, such as endorphins, oxytocin, vasopressin, and prolactin. The interaction between ovarian hormones and these neuropeptides can affect mood, memory, motor coordination, and other behaviors. Estrogen and progesterone influence multiple aspects of your brain chemistry, specifically affecting such neurotransmitters as dopamine, norepinephrine, acetylcholine, gamma aminobutyric acid, and serotonin. These are powerful mediations of emotions, mood, and behaviors. More specifically, they influence depression, irritability, anxiety, pain responsiveness, eating disorders, energy level, sex drive, and sleep. The effects of testosterone on these neurotransmitters have not been established scientifically.

Estrogen

This hormone affects numerous aspects of your premenstrual and perimenopausal experience. There are three types of estrogens produced within your body.

1. *17-Beta Estradiol.* Produced by the ovaries. The dominant estrogen, responsible for several hundred functions within the body (e.g., skin, bone, hair, brain, heart, blood vessels, etc).
2. *Estrone.* Produced by body fat and the ovaries. Also converted from estradiol and vice versa.
3. *Estriol.* Produced during pregnancy, and not measurable in nonpregnant women. Weakest of human estrogens, since it does not adequately protect bone, brain, heart, etc. Improves memory, mood, and sleep.

We will discuss other types of estrogens in the context of hormone replacement therapy in Chapter 13.

Here are some of the things that estrogen does:

- Enhances mood
- Lowers depression
- Relieves anxiety
- Raises energy level
- Enables vaginal lubrication
- Improves sleep
- Prevents hot flushes
- Regulates body temperature
- Decreases irritability
- Can improve digestion
- Reduces urinary frequency and urgency

- Can prevent urinary-tract infections
- Decreases aches and pains
- Increases the ability to concentrate
- Improves short- and long-term memory
- Enhances logical reasoning
- Shortens reaction time
- Improves motor coordination and balance
- Enhances bone-mineral density
- Improves and protects cardiovascular health
- Relieves headaches

Although this list seems to indicate that there may be many benefits of regulating your estrogen level, it is important not to conclude that you need estrogen replacement simply because you have one or more of these symptoms. The list above indicates what estrogen does inside your body, but it does not suggest that you should opt for increasing its level as a straightforward antidote to your distress. In Chapter 13, we will discuss both the benefits and possible risks of hormone replacement therapy. Before you make decisions regarding estrogen, we urge you to study that chapter.

Progesterone and Progestins

Two types of hormones, progesterone and progestins, are part of a larger group, called progestogens. At one time, these hormones were considered to be an antidote to premenstrual distress. This belief was based on a lack of understanding of the biochemistry of the menstrual cycle. Since progesterone dominates during the premenstrual, or luteal, phase of the cycle, health-care practitioners thought that adding more would be beneficial. However, more recent findings indicate that premenstrual symptoms might actually increase in intensity if you take additional progestogens during this phase. Progestogens act as an antagonist to estradiol and testosterone receptors in the brain, resulting in diminishing any effects that these hormones can produce.

Progesterone causes the sloughing off of the endometrium, thus initiating your periods. It is essential for the survival and development of a fetus. It protects against the side effects of estrogen, and it is an important precursor in the biosynthesis of the other ovarian and adrenal hormones.

Progesterone and progestins are similar but have some important differences:

1. *Progesterone.* This is the human, naturally occurring hormone produced by your ovaries and, to a much lesser extent, by your adrenal gland.

2. *Progestins.* These are manufactured hormones, many times more potent than natural progesterone. Progestins are part of the makeup of birth-control pills. They can produce more bothersome effects within your body. One type of progestin is derived from the male hormone, testosterone, and has effects more similar to testosterone than progesterone.

Progestogens can have the following effects:

- Dampened mood
- Intensified depression
- Lowered anxiety
- Decreased energy
- Lowered sex drive
- Increased irritability
- Bloating

- Water retention
- Increased appetite
- Weight gain
- Increased breast tenderness

It is clear from this list that progesterone is directly related to premenstrual and perimenopausal symptoms.

Testosterone

This is one of a group of hormones that are collectively called androgens. Androgens stimulate normal bone growth and muscle development and regulate the distribution of body fat. Most people associate testosterone with males rather than females. It is, however, a naturally occurring substance that is produced throughout the life of the ovaries, both by the ovaries themselves and the adrenal gland. The ovaries produce about one-third of your supply of androgens, in the form of testosterone. There are five androgens: testosterone, dihydrotestosterone (DHT), dehydroepiandrosterone (DHEA), dihydrotestosterone-sulphate (DHEA-S), and androstenedione. Even if your ovaries are not functioning, some testosterone is still being produced within your body by the adrenal glands. However, one of the androgens, androstenedione, decreases about 50 percent after menopause, and this results in a loss of sufficient testosterone. The presence of estradiol enables the brain to permit testosterone to produce the following effects:

- Enhances mood
- Increases energy level
- Generates a sense of well-being
- Enhances metabolic rate
- Causes sexual arousal

- Improves sexual desire
- Facilitates orgasmic functioning
- Improves problem solving
- Increases the ability to concentrate
- Improves short- and long-term memory
- Enhances logical reasoning
- Increases the ability to concentrate
- Enhances bone-mineral density

This hormone is essential for internal balance, and it can determine your level of sexual interest and satisfaction. The combination of estrogen and testosterone enhances mood and energy level more so than either does independently.

Since the adrenal gland is dynamically linked to the ovary, it is necessary to maintain health in one gland to assure that the other functions properly. Research on ovarian change from infancy through maturity indicates that (1) the size of the ovaries decreases during the thirties and (2) the ovaries can continue to secrete estradiol and testosterone, and the adrenal glands can continue to supply DHEA well past menopause. It is not clear why some women are able to maintain this pattern while others are not. During pregnancy some cells migrate from the ovaries, while other identical ones migrate from the adrenal gland, and this causes the two to interact throughout life. As you go through perimenopause, your level of androgens during the ovulatory phase of your menstrual cycle is less. Most women, for example, lose about half the capacity of their adrenal glands to produce androgens (discussed above) by ages forty to forty-four. As your ovaries function less effectively, they will supply less than sufficient levels of estrogen and testosterone. This change is likely to be accompanied by parallel loss of androgens produced by your adrenal gland.

The hormones produced by your ovaries and your adrenal gland are synchronized. There is a continuous interplay between the entire set of hormones that underlie PMS and perimenopause. Your symptoms come from the interaction of all of these hormones, your brain, the environment in which you live, and your personal psychology.

CHRONOLOGICAL VERSUS OVARIAN AGE

It is important to remember that your chronological age, or number of years since your birth, is not the same as your ovarian age. That is, you may be in your fifties and still be having regular periods, but your ovaries are functioning as though you were in your twenties or thirties. Conversely, you may be in your teens or young adulthood, with symptoms that resemble perimenopause. You have to listen to yourself and become capable of describing your symptoms accurately to health-care providers in order to determine your approximate ovarian age. These professionals may recommend the measurement of your estradiol level, FSH, testosterone, and other androgens in order to form a complete understanding of your ovarian condition. Since these measurements are not precise indicators and may fluctuate, it is important that you become acutely aware of the subtle changes that occur within your ovaries as they mature. The goal is to have your ovarian hormones in proper balance in order to avoid developing disturbing symptoms.

A NOTE ON TERMINOLOGY

Premenstrual symptoms occur within the luteal phase of your menstrual cycle. Technically, a symptom is "premenstrual" if it begins during the luteal phase and is relieved during the first one to two days after you get your period. These symptoms, discussed in detail in Chapter 7, continue through your perimenopausal stage of development. In addition, other symptoms begin during that stage. During perimenopause your premenstrual symptoms are likely to be intensified (see Chapter 8). The term *PMS*, or premenstrual syndrome, refers to the unique sets of symptoms during the luteal phase of the menstrual cycle. The term *perimenopause* refers to the developmental stage before menopause, with the menstrual cycle becoming irregular and additional symptoms emerging. In this book we use the term *premenstrual* to refer both to PMS or when you experience perimenopausal symptoms.

3

Depression, Anxiety, and Your Ovarian Hormones

Lavinia complains of "feeling down" much of the time, and her mood state is beginning to worry her friends and family. She is thirty-two, married, with two children, ages seven and nine. Her husband travels extensively as part of his job as a sales representative. Lavinia is a licensed teacher, but she has stopped working the past few years to look after their children. She talks about having frequent crying spells, which she can't seem to stop. She reports that she screams at her children. She is concerned that her anger gets out of control at times. Her energy level is much lower than it was when she was younger, and she wakes up often during the night worrying about family matters. She doesn't like how she is feeling about herself. She wants to become more in control of her moods, rather than being driven by them.

Sarah is thirty, on a fast track toward partnership in a law firm. She reports feeling anxious a lot of the time, but she does not know what makes her anxious. She worries a great deal about little things, like her clothes, completing tasks, doing things correctly, getting to meetings on time, and meeting deadlines in her work. Sarah has been in a relationship for over three years with a male lawyer at another firm, who is about her age. They have recently moved in together, and she is adjusting to living with someone for the first time in many years. She has become concerned about whether she should go ahead and have the child she wants. Her partner is pushing her to "make it legal" and to start a family right away. Sarah appears restless, and she frequently has difficulty concentrating on her work because of the pressures of her relationship.

These two scenarios illustrate that feeling depressed or anxious is a normal response that everyone experiences from time to time. These two women's emotions are not limited to responses to PMS or perimenopause, and they are not necessarily indicative of mental-health problems. Mood changes can come and go freely in everyday life. When such moods seriously interfere with your functioning, however, you may be experiencing a syndrome rather than a simple mood state. The difference is largely one of degree. If you feel "down" or "shaky," you may be able to slough off the feeling and go about your tasks normally. If you are unable to rid yourself of the feeling for a significant amount of time, the feeling may intensify. Then it can affect your thinking, behavior, and sense of self-worth.

Emotional well-being is a critical aspect of your inner life. Having the sense of being "okay" emotionally is related to being in a stable intimate relationship, having job security, perceiving that you have options, and believing that you can maintain your personal autonomy as you make life choices. If you feel trapped or limited in your options, you may make yourself vulnerable to feeling anxious and depressed. Women who are able to adapt to changes in their own and others' expectations and to changes related to the aging process tend to be stronger emotionally. Another vital concern is being able to balance work and family life so that both can nurture your sense of your world as a positive place for you.

MOOD INFLUENCERS

Some things that cause you stress come from the outside. Things happen, and you have to react. Other stressors are internal. They come from the ways you conceptualize your world and yourself, or some are rooted in changes in your physiology. Some stressors have a temporary effect, and others have lasting impact. Someone from your child's school calls and tells you that your child had a bad day. Either you simply handle this event, or you make yourself feel down about it. You are decorating your house for an upcoming party, and you discover that the plumbing in your guest bathroom isn't functioning properly. You have a deadline at work, and your computer's hard drive crashes. You are experiencing conflict over whether you should stay in a long-term, somewhat comfortable relationship with someone whom you are no longer passionate about. You notice that you are reacting to others in an impatient manner, and you are experiencing "crying jags" when watching a comedy on TV, just before you get your period. Your doctor suspects that you may be becoming diabetic, or you have just found out that your headaches are migraines. All of these stressors can evoke depression or anxiety. How you interpret these occurrences, conflicts, and changes determines the degree to which you become depressed or anxious.

Negative self-regard can lead to both depression and anxiety. We develop our sense of ourselves, or our "self-concepts," from feedback from important people in our childhood. When these people (parents, teachers, older siblings, etc.) are critical of us, make unrealistic demands, or abuse us in any way, we may develop the notion that we are not okay. Then everything that happens around us tends to validate this idea we have of ourselves. If you regard yourself in a negative manner, that is, you think that you are limited, unintelligent, unattractive, or weak, you have a tendency not to act self-confidently. This can create a cycle that is sometimes referred to as a self-fulfilling prophecy. You don't even try to become chair of the committee, and if you do, you act so tentatively that others don't choose you, proving what you already know about yourself—that you are somehow undesirable. Positive self-regard, on the other hand, includes knowing and accepting your limitations as well as your strengths. You behave proactively, working toward achievable goals that you have set for yourself. Looking at yourself positively has important implications for avoiding the debilitating effects of depression and anxiety.

> *Carolyn* says, "I don't know whether I have PMS or not. Every month I get more depressed and angry. I scream at my family. I'm even depressed at work, and it's obvious. My husband thinks that I 'have it.' The last two months, my memory just left me before I got my period. I forget where I put things. While driving I forget where I'm going." She has been noticing weight gain, feeling bloated, and having breast tenderness just before she gets her period. "Food cravings are a problem in general for me, and before my period I just can't stay away from chocolate and desserts."

Dolores reports, "I never had problems with PMS before I had my son. It's been getting worse the past few years." She describes having a lot of anxiety, with occasional feelings of panic. She sometimes gets these panic attacks in grocery stores, crossing bridges, and being in open spaces—always when she is by herself. Her impulse is to run in order to get away from these feelings. The attacks are more frequent and more intense just before she gets her periods. She is easily distracted, and she tends to "take things personally" when things happen around her. During the past year she has had a number of hot flushes, for the first time, and her periods are not as regular as they used to be. "My friends tell me that I'm just not like myself any more. They tell me that I am not as outgoing as I have been, and they worry about me."

Harriett had her first child six weeks ago. The delivery was uneventful. She describes herself as being okay during pregnancy, with her moods being stable and positive. Since giving birth, however, she has been experiencing many crying spells and being fearful of hurting the baby or doing something wrong. She worries about whether she will be a good mother. She is not getting enough sleep, since she breast-feeds the child several times during the night. She says, "I feel like my world is caving in. I'm just not able to function. My husband is paying more attention to the baby than he is to me. I don't want to go out of the house. I have always been a social and upbeat person. I don't understand what's happening to me."

These three vignettes show that during your ovarian life span there are three times when you are most vulnerable to experiencing difficulties with depression and anxiety. These occur in accordance with ovarian-related conditions—PMS, postpartum, and perimenopause. Two additional ovarian-related conditions—pregnancy and postmenopause—have significantly less chance of bringing on depression and anxiety. Postpartum depression or anxiety, however, is quite prevalent. This is a time when the ovarian hormones can fluctuate rapidly and erratically. The more your ovarian hormones fluctuate the more you are likely to have depression and anxiety interfere with your normal activities.

During PMS, postpartum, and perimenopause, your levels of estrogen, progesterone, and testosterone change both in rate and level. These changes result in corresponding changes in your brain chemistry, affecting your mood, thinking, and behavior. During pregnancy your ovarian hormones are three times higher than normal for you, and during postmenopause they are the lowest, unless you are on hormone replacement therapy. During both pregnancy and postmenopause your ovarian hormones are the most stable, consistently high or low, and they have the least likelihood of presenting you with mood alterations such as depression or anxiety.

With regard to PMS and perimenopause there are three patterns of experiencing depression or anxiety:

1. Your depression and anxiety are not related directly to your menstrual cycle and are present almost all the time. This condition may require that you receive psychotherapeutic and medical treatment. (See Chapter 13.)
2. The depression and anxiety symptoms occur in a rhythmic, recurrent fashion during the luteal phase of your cycle. This pattern can appear both during PMS and perimenopause.

3. The mood disorder of depression or anxiety becomes exacerbated when the ovarian hormones fluctuate, such as they do in PMS and perimenopause.

The rhythms of the menstrual cycle have a marked connection to your emotional state. The risk for developing mood changes or a mood disorder that requires treatment intensifies as your cycle changes and your ovaries age. PMS symptoms commonly become more intensified in the late thirties to mid-forties, often accompanied by a new onset of depression and anxiety. The link seems to be related to the instability of ovarian hormone production, which affects brain neurotransmitters, resulting in a destabilization of mood-regulating mechanisms. When ovarian-hormone changes during your menstrual cycle cause the serotonin level to lower within your brain, you are more vulnerable to developing depressive and anxiety symptoms. Declining estrogen during midlife, corresponding to perimenopause, also seems to be correlated with higher vulnerability to depression and anxiety disorders.

Your experiences during midlife are likely to be the most stressful of any time in your development other than puberty. During puberty hormones emerge as a significant determiner of one's sense of well-being, yet young women lack the experiences with which to compare this new reality. The appearance of secondary sex characteristics brings excitement, embarrassment, and concerns about beginning womanhood, meanwhile others may still be relating to you as though you were a child. Being propelled into sexuality, menstruation, and reproductive capability can generate an array of emotional reactions. During your mid-thirties to mid-forties the factors that put pressure on you are decidedly different. You may be struggling with teenagers or young children or wondering whether you really want to have children. You may be coping with changes in your relationship with a significant other.

You may be "topped out" in your career or are returning to work or school. It is not uncommon to reflect on your mortality since you are aware of no longer being "bulletproof." In addition, you may be self-conscious about changes in your own body, such as wrinkles, sagging, weight gain, loss of stamina, and change in the "youthful look" to one of maturity. When you put this all together, you can see how your vulnerability to anxiety and depression is highest at this age.

What Are Mood Disorders?

Mood disorders, sometimes referred to as affective disorders, are ongoing emotional states that interfere significantly with your daily functioning. Mood disorders are most commonly related to depression or anxiety, and some women experience both. You may be temporarily sad, "down," or tense, but this does not indicate a mood disorder.

These mood disorders may or may not be connected to your menstrual cycle. If you are prone to a mood disorder, going through ovarian change may precipitate depression or anxiety to the degree that you need psychotherapeutic assistance. If you are already experiencing a mood disorder, PMS or perimenopause can intensify the condition.

Your feelings become problematic when they last for some time and get in the way of your regular routines. A transient feeling may be unpleasant, but it may be nothing more than a feeling of the moment. It could also be a symptom of something else that you have to cope with, such as physical illness, grief over a significant loss, or an indication that you are dreading something undesirable. If you find yourself depressed or anxious for a prolonged period of time, however, you may be suffering from a mood disorder, and you may need some form of treatment, such as those discussed in Chapter 13.

Depression

Clinical depression causes difficulty for about one out of every four adults sometime during their lifetimes. Depression can be considered a mood state, a syndrome, or simply a symptom. How it is considered depends in large part on its severity and the degree to which it is interfering with ordinary functioning. The risk of death from depression is higher than that of breast cancer. So, it is important to consider the seriousness of this disorder.

The most common factors among people who are clinically depressed are prior depressive episodes, a family history of depression, being female, ovarian hormonal fluctuations, and high levels of stress or trauma. Both hysterectomy (removal of the uterus) and tubal ligation (severing the fallopian tubes) cause less blood to flow to the ovaries. This can result in less production of ovarian hormones and bring on depression. Partial oophorectomy, or the removal of one ovary, can also decrease the amount of hormones available and leave the woman open to depression. Complete (bilateral) oophorectomy means that no ovarian hormones will be produced, and this can raise the likelihood of depression, particularly in young women.

There are three major depression syndromes: Major Depressive Disorder, Dysthymic Disorder, and Bipolar Disorder. Each of these clusters of symptoms includes the following:

- Sadness
- A persistent down mood
- Loss of interest in normally pleasurable activities
- Changes in sleep patterns, appetite, and sexual desire
- Poor concentration
- Narrowing of attention span

- Thoughts of suicide
- Feelings of worthlessness and inadequacy
- Hopelessness
- Fatigue

Women who experience these symptoms in an intense and ongoing way, at levels that interfere with social and occupational functioning, are likely to be suffering from depression.

Major Depressive Disorder: Single or Recurrent Episode. This condition exists when your symptoms last two weeks or more. Of people over age eighteen, about 6 percent have this disorder at least once in their lives. Most of these are women, since the prevalence among them of Major Depressive Disorder is 7 percent, as opposed to only 3 percent of men. In about 2 percent of people, this disorder lasts for at least one month. The duration of an untreated major depression is usually six to nine months, with a 50 percent chance that it will recur. Having this disorder can be debilitating. You feel "blue" most of the time, your energy level is very low, you may cry uncontrollably, your interest in what would be normally pleasurable for you is low, and you find yourself being easily irritated and distracted. You tend to "take things out on" other people. You may have thoughts of death, suicide, and what life is all about. You may not feel like eating normally, and you can have trouble falling asleep at night. You may be experiencing significant depression for the first time (single episode), or you may have the condition several times (recurrent episode). Major depression is a serious condition, and it usually requires both psychotherapy and medical attention.

Dysthymic Disorder. In this condition, depressive symptoms are experienced for two years or more. Women have this disorder more than men do—4 percent compared to 2 percent. These symptoms may be experienced for long periods yet go unrecognized. You may, however, become aware that something is wrong. You may come to feel that you are alone and "stuck." Everything is a "drag." Life becomes a chore. You may begin to eat compulsively as an only pleasure. Your sexual desire may be very low. Everything is an effort to do. You may think that everyone feels like you. When you do get relief through treatment, you may discover that your way of viewing your own life suddenly changes. You may gain an enhanced appreciation of living.

Bipolar Disorder. This condition is sometimes referred to as *manic depressive.* A person with Bipolar Disorder has both depressive and manic symptoms. You might have periods of significant sadness, followed by episodes of having a very high mood. You might be extremely low for a period of time and then notice a rapid acceleration in your general emotional makeup, which persists for another period. Your symptoms may be the opposite of those listed above. This disorder is equally common in women and men (about 1 percent each) throughout their lifetimes, but women experience rapidly alternating Bipolar Disorder more often than men do.

Depression hits women significantly more often than men. This inordinate prevalence among women may be related to numerous factors, such as genetics, stress, socioeconomic status, traumatic events, use of stimulants and hallucinogens, use and abuse of alcohol and drugs, and ovarian hormone makeup and its interaction with neurotransmitters. (Although alcoholism is five times higher among men, women with this affliction often experience much more depression and anxiety.) Any combination of these factors can cause biochemical changes, leading to a depressive condition. Depression can also result from chronic medical conditions, such as complications of hypothyroidism and diabetes.

Sometimes people confuse depression with exhaustion, burnout, or fatigue. You can experience a change in energy level, and it could be temporary or an established pattern. Temporary changes in energy level can be one indicator of depression, more symptoms should manifest before being diagnosed as depressed. Your level of energy may drop temporarily from some external event, such as your cat becoming ill and feeling sad about it. You may "bounce back" without sustaining the mood. If you are experiencing prolonged physical fatigue, you may be suffering primarily from dietary insufficiency, heavy exercise, an external crisis, or a negative physiological condition. Feeling depressed may be a secondary effect of such causes.

Depression is one of over sixty symptoms of the syndrome termed "burnout." You are "burning out" when your ability to function is significantly below what is normal for you over a period of time. The most common symptoms are job-related stress, having lots of unfinished business and "loose ends," worry about personal finances, and impatience. Your motivation may get lost, your energy level may drop, and you may lose interest in what is normally interesting to you. As a result, you may be taking away the activities in your life that sustain you. You may be experiencing some aspects of depression, but you may be primarily suffering from the burnout syndrome.

Anxiety

Like depression, anxiety can be considered a mood state, a syndrome, or simply a symptom. If you are experiencing tension, it may come from ordinary events. You may also experience a level of excitement, like "butterflies" or the heady feeling of falling in love. You may feel a temporary rush when you attempt something that you have never done before. Normally women rebound from these feelings quickly. If the emotions are sustained for a long period, they may become troublesome. You are said to be clinically anxious when you are experiencing fear or dread to a degree that interferes with your ability to do your normal activities. Your concern may be general, or "free-floating," or it may be highly specific, as in the various phobias. Your anxiety may come in the form of a "panic attack." Your ovarian-hormone balance can determine the level and duration of your anxiety. In addition, feeling anxious may be a warning sign that you have some medical situation that needs attention.

In ovarian-related conditions in which anxiety is the predominant mood, the physiological changes that may occur follow this sequence:

1. Your estrogen level lowers, as in the premenstrual phase of your cycle.
2. The change in estradiol level signals the brain.
3. The neurotransmitter serotonin drops, the neurotransmitter norepinephrine increases, and the neuropeptide endorphin drops.
4. You may experience anxiety, with such symptoms as tension, irritability, sleep disturbances, sweating or chilling sensations, "butterflies" in the stomach, diarrhea, palpitations, heart pounding, increased heart rate, increased blood pressure, clammy skin, dizziness, feeling out of control, headaches, shortness of breath, worrying, repetitive thoughts, and flashbacks to a traumatic event.

The three most common anxiety disorders are the Generalized Anxiety Disorder, Panic Disorder (with or without Agoraphobia), and Specific or Social Phobia.

Generalized Anxiety Disorder. People who are diagnosed with this disorder have excessive worry that occurs more days than not for at least six months. It may be focused on a number of different activities or events, such as work, school, or home life. People can have a lot of worry in relation to having a history of panic attacks, phobic experiences, physical complaints, or serious illness. Anxiety is the most common undesirable reaction to stress. The disorder may be related to the use of prescribed medications or other substance use. This disorder affects women and men equally.

A complex of the following symptoms characterizes this syndrome:

- Excessive anxiety and worry
- Restlessness or feeling "on edge"
- Being easily fatigued
- Having difficulty concentrating or having the mind go blank
- Irritability
- Muscle tension
- Sleep disturbance

Panic Disorder (with or without Agoraphobia). This condition is often missed or misdiagnosed. It can lead to social isolation or phobias. A panic episode occurs in a brief time period, in which one is faced with intense fear or discomfort, coming from a combination of the following symptoms:

- Heart palpitations
- Sweating
- Trembling or shaking
- Sensations of shortness of breath or smothering
- Feelings of choking
- Chest pain or discomfort
- Nausea or abdominal distress

- Feeling dizzy, unsteady, lightheaded, or faint
- Feelings of unreality or being detached from oneself
- Fear of losing control or going crazy
- Fear of dying
- Numbness or tingling sensations
- Chills or hot flushes

The diagnosis requires the presence of fear or discomfort and at least four of the above symptoms. If the person is also experiencing Agoraphobia, feeling that you are in a situation from which you cannot escape or in which you fear having an embarrassing panic attack, the fears involve situations such as the following:

- Being outside the home
- Being in a crowd or standing in a line
- Being on a bridge
- Traveling in a bus, train, or automobile

A person who is prone to a Panic Disorder with Agoraphobia avoids these situations or else endures them with marked distress, or they require the presence of a trusted companion.

Specific or Social Phobia. Both these phobias are marked by persistent, intense fear. Specific phobias are centered on specific objects or situations, such as flying, heights, animals, insects, and so on. A person with Social Phobia fears being scrutinized by unfamiliar people in social or performance situations. The symptoms are the same as those of the Generalized Anxiety Disorder.

Research on Social Phobia indicates that it may occur in adolescence, associated with parental over-protectiveness. Females and males are equally affected. About 7 percent of the general population suffer from some phobia, and this is not connected with a history of family mental illness or a history of having the same phobia within the immediate family.

Although we have discussed depression and anxiety separately, they are often part of a woman's total experience as she copes with life changes and the aging of her ovarian function. There are no simple ways of separating the two intense emotional states since they can co-exist in response to a great variety of stimuli.

Depression and anxiety can deplete your energy and make life decidedly unpleasant, not only for you but also for the people around you. When you couple these two maladies with PMS or perimenopause, you may be challenged to cope. In Chapter 13 we will discuss several types of treatment to work yourself out of these conditions if you develop them. Both depression and anxiety are treatable. When you take personal responsibility for improving your moods, you may improve your ovarian condition as well. You do not have to "suffer through" feeling bad all the time. Advances in psychotherapy, medicine, and alternative treatments offer hope for all women who suffer from these conditions.

AM I LOSING
MY MIND?

fluctuations in ovarian hormones can affect your ability to
think clearly, concentrate, remember things, and generally perform mental tasks. Both PMS and perimenopause take a toll on
your cognitive functioning. Just before your period you may experience a number of symptoms that show this interference with
your thinking. In this chapter we will explore the concept of cognition, or how your brain processes information, the effects of sex
hormones, how your thinking can change during your menstrual
cycle, effects of aging, and environmental influences.

Consider the cases of Cassandra, Kathy, and Melissa. They
represent common experiences that are directly related to PMS
and perimenopause.

> *Cassandra* is twenty-two, a senior in the university.
> She says, "It's like I'm outside my body. I'm doing

things I can't believe. My boyfriend showed up for our lunch date fifteen minutes late, and I felt sure that I had caused it. People say things, and I take them personally. I overreact. Sometimes I can't seem to get myself organized to go to class. I'm really afraid I'm losing it."

Kathy is twenty-six, a checkout sales person in a department store. She says, "I just don't feel good about myself. I doubt my own worth these days. I feel like other people know that I'm not okay. I get distracted easily, and this is getting in the way of my work. I even find myself sometimes unable to make change correctly."

Melissa is forty-seven, and her three children have left home. She owns and operates a boutique. She says, "I sometimes have trouble listening to people. I even forget the names of my regular customers occasionally, and it seems to be happening more frequently these days. I seem to be muddled, and I'm just not as sharp as I need to be to run this business."

Women often say that there are times when they do not think clearly. If you are premenstrual or perimenopausal, you may be able to identify with these statements:

I'm at a party, and I can't recall a good friend's name.

I forgot whether I mailed my rent check.

I seem to be in a fog constantly.

Sometimes I can't seem to solve easy problems.

I can't seem to keep my priorities straight.

I was driving to see my doctor, and I forgot the way.

I was about to tell someone my telephone number, and I drew a blank.

Things are coming at me too fast for me to react.

I am often in the middle of an important meeting, and I am mentally cooking my dinner.

I tend to forget my kids' birthdays—something I never did before.

I hear the words, but they don't compute.

I have difficulty laying out all the steps needed to accomplish work tasks, so I feel chaotic.

Did I close the garage door?

I have to juggle the schedules of the kids, my work, and time with my spouse, and nowadays I can't seem to find a logical solution.

All these statements are normal for some people some of the time, but they are all worrisome when they suddenly begin to occur more frequently and interfere with your daily functioning.

Many aspects of our life experiences affect how we think, and women have particular concern about the effects of the phases of their menstrual cycles and their ovarian-hormonal fluctuations. Other things that can influence thinking may be other physiological conditions, such as thyroid disorders, diabetes, neurological diseases, cardiovascular problems, etc. In addition, effectiveness in thinking can be negatively affected by mood, stress, substance use, sleeping disorders, diet, and various medications.

COGNITION

Scientists use the term *cognition* to refer to the states and processes that the brain uses to take in and manipulate information and to communicate effectively with the outside world. The major dimensions of cognition are perceptual speed and accuracy, memory (short-, medium-, and long-term; verbal and spatial), attention, focusing, concentration, organization, reasoning, and reaction time. Other dimensions of cognition include verbal fluency and expression. Both PMS and perimenopause affect all of these skills. Your thinking is likely to be influenced negatively by the fluctuation of your ovarian hormones as you go through your menstrual cycles and as your ovaries age.

There are dominant "styles" of receiving, processing, and communicating in reaction to information. Research indicates that about two-thirds of us, both female and male, are primarily visual in taking in information, with a secondary preference for auditory (hearing) and a third emphasis on kinesthetic (touch) modes. Then we strongly tend to use what is termed *parallel processing* (thinking about several things at once) rather than *serial processing* (thinking about things one at a time). Finally, we strongly tend to use visual modes of communicating, using auditory and kinesthetic modes to a lesser degree.

Sex Hormones and Cognition

Gender differences in cognition can be somewhat attributed to sex hormones that affect the development of fetuses. The sex hormones include estrogen, progesterone, and the androgens, which are produced by both the ovaries and the adrenal gland. Both estrogen and the androgens influence the brain structure and functioning, thus determining in large part the cognition of the individual after birth. In other words, female fetuses, exposed to higher levels of estrogen and lower levels of androgens than are male fetuses can develop more pronounced right-brain dominance, with enhanced verbal abilities, perceptual speed and accuracy, rote memory, and fine-motor skills. Conversely, male fetuses, with less estrogen and higher levels of androgens available, tend to have superior spatial skills, quantitative ability and mathematical reasoning, and gross-motor strength, with left-brain dominance.

Hormone replacement therapy, which we discuss in Chapter 13, can affect these differences in cognitive skills, but the basic "programming" will remain as it was at birth. Studies have shown that the use of estrogen that is supplied externally can result in improvements in both mood and cognition. It either maintains or enhances verbal abilities in women, as well as improving both short- and long-term verbal memory, enhancing logical reasoning, decreasing reaction time, and improving attention and focusing ability. Replacing estrogen can have a protective effect for older women, increasing blood flow to the brain, helping to prevent cerebral vascular disease (mild strokes), and lowering the incidence of Alzheimer's disease, dementia, and intellectual decline. Testosterone replacement therapy can benefit women by enhancing logical reasoning and short- and long-term memory. Replacing both estrogen and testosterone can optimize the beneficial effects of each.

Several studies have compared women who have gone through the menopause with those who still have ovarian functioning. Differences in the cognitive functioning of these groups of women appear to be primarily in the areas of memory for learned information, verbal memory, reaction time, articulatory and fine-motor skills, spatial relations, and memory for proper names (not for words). In all of these studies, women who have normal ovarian functioning scored higher. A woman who no longer has a menstrual cycle, or who is having less frequent ones, may begin to wonder whether she is "losing her mind." What is likely happening is that the lack of ovarian hormones is causing her to feel "spacey," slow, ungrounded, and impatient with her inability to think clearly and remain organized.

Since sex hormones influence the development of brain functioning, they also affect communications between females and males. If you perceive the world artistically, for example, and your significant other is a "by-the-numbers" sort of person, the two of you may experience frequent miscommunications. A similar mismatch may occur between two females or between two males whose cognitive functioning has been significantly influenced by different levels of the sex hormones during gestation. There is evidence that the sex hormones of the developing fetus determine the dominance of the two hemispheres of the brain. A "masculine" profile of gonadal hormones tends strongly to produce left-brain dominance, which features analytic and spatial relations, while a "feminine" profile results in right-brain competency in intuition, nonverbal processing, and verbal ability. Up until puberty, the differences in cognitive functioning between females and males are less apparent. When your ovarian hormones begin changing cyclically, your cognitive functioning is likely to become affected, and differences between you and males may become more obvious. When your ovarian hormones begin to fluctuate unpredictably, as in perimenopause, your brain may seem to fail you at inopportune times.

There is an old joke that illustrates the point. A wife says to her husband during breakfast, "Honey, I love you." He replies, "Let's begin by defining our terms." Later during the meal, she complains, "Can't we have just one argument without using logic?" These two people may be acting out differences in how their cognition works, and this can cause difficulties in the relationship. If the wife is premenstrual or perimenopausal, these differences may be accentuated by her changing levels of ovarian hormones.

Cognition and the Menstrual Cycle

During the phases of your menstrual cycle there are important changes in your cognitive functioning. Research indicates that during the follicular phase (see Chapter 2) you are apt to have higher verbal fluency and memory and lower performance on tasks that require visual/spatial ability. During the luteal phase you may experience a number of cognitive/attentional phenomena, including loss of focus, inability to reason normally, difficulty thinking clearly, difficulty making decisions, slower reaction time, and forgetfulness. The menstrual cycle seems to have little or no effect on your general level of intellectual ability, however.

Numerous researchers have also commented on a lack of difference between the phases of the menstrual cycle and the quality of cognition. In other words, among women who have periods, there appears to be no difference between when they are in the follicular and luteal phases, when their estrogen levels are highest and lowest. It may be that the difference between these two phases is subtler than the difference between women who have and do not have ovarian function. Postmenopausal women, who have little or no natural estrogen, suffer marked losses in cognition. It may also be that both progesterone and testosterone levels, which decline premenstrually and drop to negligible levels after menopause, have effects on cognition.

These studies produced another interesting, consistent, and somewhat surprising finding. There appears to be little or no relationship between temporary mood states and cognitive functioning. For example, if you are feeling sad or anxious when you are premenstrual, you may still be able to process information effectively and continue to keep track of the activities that you need to engage in during that time. If you are perimenopausal, your hormones may be fluctuating more significantly. In the luteal phase you may have to work harder to overcome the effects of mood swings in order to keep your cognitive functioning adequate.

Effects of Aging

It is commonly observed that cognitive functioning changes as we age. Numerous aging processes can cause deterioration in our mental efficiency. The most obvious for women are changes in ovarian and adrenal functioning, affecting gonadal hormones. These hormones may play a protective role against age-related deterioration in some cognitive abilities. Other aging processes that can affect your thinking apparatus are normal changes in brain chemistry and structure and lessening physical reactivity, which negatively affects perceptual speed and reaction time.

Since Alzheimer's disease is four times more common in elderly women than in men of the same age, it is natural for women to be concerned about it. If dementia (deterioration of cognitive functioning) is caught early, the treatment effect is more pronounced. Estrogen plays an important role in retaining your memory, and your natural supply of estrogen declines with age. Research is showing that women with Alzheimer's disease and other forms of dementia respond positively to estrogen replacement therapy. Estrogen increases blood flow to the brain, and this may contribute to the improvements that have been observed.

The aging process involves changes in our self-concepts. As we progress from childhood through adult maturity, we modify how we see ourselves. Body changes cause us to think about ourselves differently, thereby affecting how we perceive and react to the world around us. Others alter how they react to us; in turn, our information processing, reasoning, and assumptions mediate how we relate to them.

Environmental Influences on Cognition

Not all brain activity is determined at birth. How we think and behave also changes as a result of the environments we grow up in and encounter as adults. The environment in which pregnant women live can even affect fetuses. Stress, medications, drugs, nutrition, climate, medical or psychiatric conditions—all these can influence the levels of the sex hormones to which fetuses are exposed, resulting in variations in brain formation.

After birth an individual is exposed to a large number of additional environmental factors, such as family and culture. Sex-role stereotyping, for example, varies across cultures. In some male-dominated societies, females are "taught" to be inferior to males in mathematics, logic, scientific pursuits, and other mental abilities. Other family influences can condition mental abilities. Female children in families that reward intellectual achievement regardless of gender may develop significant abilities to engage in a broad range of cognitive challenges.

Communication is a central cognitive activity, and it often reflects the effects of upbringing, adult life experiences, and basic brain functioning. Failures in communication can result not only from our foundational mental "programming" but also from how we are nurtured as children, how others treat us as adults, and by our sense of our selves.

RATIONALITY AND HORMONES

The research on the relationships between cognitive functioning and sex hormones has not adequately taken into account the concept of irrationality. Here are some statements like those that women often make while they are premenstrual.

The party was a real flop. I guess I blew it.

You said you liked my dress. You didn't say anything about my new hair style.

My boss told me that I did a good job but I could still improve. What's the matter with me that I didn't do it right the first time?

I ought to feel good all the time.

I should know how to handle my frustrations better.

I should be able to make my husband happy all the time.

I need to be available whenever my kids need me.

I don't need any time for myself because my family is what's important.

Since everything is metabolized as glucose, it doesn't matter what I eat.

If I just wish it away, it won't bother me.

If I could just get the time to take leisurely walks, my PMS symptoms should disappear.

If I eat right, my cycles will eventually straighten out.

There are flaws in each of these statements. Being irrational includes not being aware of thinking in an illogical manner. If you find yourself thinking in terms of should, ought, must, always, if only, yes but, you may be thinking irrationally. Just before your period you may discover that you "personalize" things, take responsibility for everything that happens around you, overgeneralize, overreact, and make poor connections between facts and conclusions. You may also engage in more arguments with those close to you at home and work, and you may perceive others as not supportive of you.

We all distort and deny what others say, but some women report that this tendency is more intense premenstrually and during perimenopause. In other words, clinical experience with such women leads to the speculation that there is a real connection between hormonal fluctuations and the ability to use rational thought processes reliably. Estrogen levels are lowest premenstrually, and they fluctuate significantly during the perimenopause. It seems likely that these occurrences can increase any tendency toward irrationality. It may also be the case that lowered androgens affect your rationality.

If you are premenstrual or perimenopausal with fluctuating ovarian hormones, you may have more of a tendency than usual to think and behave irrationally. The first step in improving this condition is to become aware of the danger of making mental errors. You need to debate the assumptions and conclusions you make and apply tests of logic to them.

So, Am I Really Losing My Mind?

If you have at least a part of one ovary that is active, you can expect fluctuations in your cognitive functioning during your menstrual cycle. If you are prone to severe PMS, the cognitive symptoms are likely to be more dramatic. Being perimenopausal means that you may experience cognitive/attentional symptoms for longer periods, more intensely, and more frequently.

You may become concerned that you are "losing your mind." The term does not, of course, refer to a clinical process. Losing contact with reality, having lasting delusions, hallucinating, feeling seriously disconnected from self or others are not caused by ovarian functioning. As your ovaries age, you may notice changes in how you think and process information. Observing such is a first step in obtaining appropriate help. Hormone replacement therapy may not be regulating your cognitive processes and may be off target, so you may need changes in dosage, type, or both. Treatments for cognitive difficulties will be discussed in Chapter 13.

Living Through a Continuum

"The trouble with the turning points in life
is that there are no green arrows."

—Anonymous

The only things constant in our lives are change and our basic personalities. When we consider the thousands of changes we have undergone since birth, we begin to notice that only change is constant. Our lives are fluid, and we continuously experience the ebbs and flows of life events and physical changes. Although our sense of selves shifts during our maturing processes, we are basically the same persons that we were in childhood. At the core we are remarkably stable, while we adapt to the many events, conflicting demands, and changes that we experience while aging. We choose new directions for ourselves in response to these factors, and we propel ourselves (or are swept) into the future.

Maggie is forty-eight and perimenopausal. She is experiencing hot flushes, night sweats, moodiness, and other new symptoms that she never had as a younger woman. She is having less predictable periods, and she is considering whether to begin hormone replacement therapy. She is less fulfilled in her marriage than before, and she seems to have "topped out" in her career. She is questioning, "What's it all about? Where do I go from here?"

Her daughter *Angie* is twenty-two, and she has moderate PMS symptoms. Her career is beginning to "take off," and she is enjoying dating a number of young men. Her premenstrual discomfort centers on mood changes, bloating, and some difficulty with concentration. She is learning how to plan her activities around the luteal phase of her cycle. She moved into her first apartment about a year ago, and she talks with Maggie almost daily.

"Mother, I think I'm about to get my period. I feel down, and I am forgetting things again. Just this morning, I lost my train of thought in an important business meeting. It was really embarrassing."

"Just you wait, honey, that may happen to you a lot when you get my age. There are days when I just can't seem to get organized at all."

"I've got a date coming up tonight with a new guy, and I just hope that I'll be okay. I'm afraid that I might get emotional for no reason at all."

"I understand that completely. Sometimes I cry without being able to stop. What I've learned to do is to close myself in my room for a while and block out the world. I learned that from your grandmother. We never talked about periods or anything like that, but I did notice that there were several times when her emotions would get out of control, and she would lock herself in her room."

"Are you suggesting that I try that? Life's kinda short to run away like that."

"The difference is that we are talking about it. Maybe we can come up with something different for you. It may be that your job stress is getting to you."

"I've thought a lot about that lately. I really like my work, but sometimes I feel exhausted by it. I can't seem to walk away from it. I even think about it sometimes while I'm on a date."

"We are worriers in our family. I remember your grandmother worrying a lot about us. She would tell stories about waking in the middle of the night, not being able to go back to sleep, worrying about getting us ready for school and whether she could get all the chores done the next day. You could see it on her face."

"I guess what you're telling me is that this has been going on for generations in our family. I'm pretty optimistic, though, about handling my premenstrual changes and the advancement of my career."

"It's all a learning process. At my age, though, I'm beginning to search for new directions in my life. My body is changing, my menstrual cycles are more different than they've ever been, and I just try to maintain some kind of perspective on knowing that there are solutions available for what feels chaotic to me. My doctor says that I may be helped a lot by exercising more, changing my diet, and considering hormone replacement. If I do all that, my hope is that I will feel better about myself."

This scenario illustrates some of the changes that women experience during their lives. Sometimes the most dramatic changes are predictable, since women tend to pass on myths, practices, information, and support to the next generation. The extent to which PMS and perimenopausal difficulties are inherited or learned will undoubtedly be debated for many years to come. It is clear, however, that if mothers and daughters talk with each other openly about such matters, they can be both resourceful to each other in meeting the challenges of aging. Access to grandmothers can be instructive as well. Their experiences may be hidden by older taboos, but their premenstrual behavior can offer clues to women about their own symptoms. Life today is, of course, more complex and places new stresses on women than their mothers and grandmothers may have faced, but grandmothers can often pass on wisdom that later generations can use.

A JAGGED LINE

Women have more rhythmic patterns in their life occurrences than men, since they have menstrual and reproductive cycles. They also have more "discontinuities," or interruptions, in their orderly development. This means that women have to adjust frequently to new realities, such as beginning menses, becoming pregnant, going through childbirth and lactation, coping with premenstrual "ups and downs," and living through the transition from perimenopause to menopause.

As we progress through the continuum of time, we gradually unfold. While we think of time as linear, the reality of female development is more like a jagged line, with ups, downs, ins, and outs. Our potentials, interests, competencies, needs, and personal values become more apparent to us as we discover them in reaction to the world around us and the changes within our bodies. Many people who have studied these processes have indicated that there are somewhat predictable life stages through which we develop. Women not only grow in terms of their psychological development but also in terms of their ovarian functioning and corresponding ovarian-related conditions—PMS and perimenopause.

Life stages "ain't what they used to be." Women are living longer than ever before, and this causes shifts in expectations about the length of these life stages. Here are some examples of development that are unique to today's woman:

- Girls begin menstruation as early as ten years of age.
- Some women are having irregular menstrual cycles in their thirties, after having regular ones.
- Other women are having regular cycles until their late fifties.
- There is a growing incidence of having the first child in the late thirties and early forties.
- Use of *in vitro* insemination during the late thirties and forties has increased.
- There is an increased use of fertility-assistance services during the late thirties and forties.
- Grandmothers in their fifties and third parties are hosting embryos for women who are in their late thirties and forties.
- The use of "surrogate" or donor eggs is more prevalent among women in their late thirties into the fifties, either having the surrogate mother bear the child or using her eggs for impregnation.
- There is a shift in careers from in-home to external employment in the forties and fifties.
- There is an increase in abortions during the forties.

- Hormone replacement therapy for PMS and perimenopause is more prevalent.
- There is an increase in emphasis on career
  advancement.
- Some women begin careers in their sixties.
- Many women are placing more emphasis on planning for aging and retirement.
- There is increased time pressure in balancing work,
  family, fitness, and personal interests, especially in
  the thirties and forties.
- There is an increased emphasis on life style and its
  effects on health.

These shifts mean that women are living very different lives
than past generations. What was the norm for females yesterday is
no longer "normal." We have to construct our own notions and
develop our own models of what our life paths are and how we
want our futures to emerge.

Female Life Stages

For the purposes of this book, we will restrict ourselves to considering life stages in terms of both psychological and ovarian development, with their corresponding effects on PMS and
perimenopause. Table 5-1 shows the highlights of how a woman
develops through the major life stages.

While most women's experiences might be reflected in this
chart, life is not a smooth transition through predictable phases.
Some women experience shorter and longer times for these stages.
For example, a woman in her late twenties who is married and
wants to get pregnant may experience fertility problems. She is

achievement-oriented, and her career is taking a good shape. She is taking a fertility medication, with some emotional side effects, such as increased irritability and sadness. Each time she gets her period, it reminds her of her infertility, and this intensifies mood problems. Her PMS is not stabilized because of the fertility medication, and her infertility problems are more typical of women in middle adulthood.

Another example is a woman in her late thirties who has been experiencing mood shifts premenstrually, and has noticed that these "jags" have been intensifying. If she is also beginning to have irregularities in menstrual cycle and flow, with periodic heat waves that progress into hot flushes and cause sleep disturbances, she may be moving into perimenopause much earlier than anticipated. Women in middle adulthood are often pushing for career advancement which often causes them to encounter personal and organizational limitations and prejudices. In this stage many women reassess their total life situation because feelings of stagnation and discontent. They also face the loss of youthful illusions. During this time menstrual cycles tend to be regular, but slowly decline in length and frequency when there is more ovarian instablility. Ovarian hormone production fluctuates greatly. During the early part of this stage women tend to be more aware of their emotional and cognitive premenstrual symptoms. Later, premenstrual symptoms tend to intensify.

In utero. The fetus's developmental task is to become capable of living outside the womb. Before birth you are given the basic "wiring" that partly determines your fundamental personality structure. The foundation of your psycho-neuroendocrine combination takes shape. This becomes the blueprint for both physical and psychological development after birth. As we pointed out in Chapter 2, the development of the ovaries includes all of the follicles and ova that a female will have throughout her lifetime.

Table 5-1

LIFE STAGE	PSYCHOLOGICAL DEVELOPMENT	OVARIAN DEVELOPMENT	PMS AND PERIMENOPAUSE
In utero	Inheriting predisposition to personality	Creation of ovaries, follicles, and lifetime supply of ova	No symptoms
Infancy and early childhood 0–8	Attachment and bonding; development of trust in others; beginning sense of self as different from others; development of gender identity; rapid learning	Slow maturation of ovarian and pituitary functions	No symptoms
Late Childhood 8–12	Ability to interact effectively with the environment, including the ability to complete activities; creation of a set of personal values; developing peer relations	Ovarian-pituitary interaction, with hormone secretion	No symptoms
Puberty Varies widely, usually 11–15	Heightened erotic development, with sexual desire and arousal; increased self-consciousness regarding body changes	Secondary-sex characteristics triggered by testosterone; onset of menses; capability of reproduction	First experience of premenstrual symptoms

Table 5-1 *continued*

LIFE STAGE	PSYCHOLOGICAL DEVELOPMENT	OVARIAN DEVELOPMENT	PMS AND PERIMENOPAUSE
Adolescence 12–18	Completing a sense of identity; resolving dependency vs. autonomy issues; facing challenges regarding intimacy; developing ability to fall in love	Ovarian-pituitary interaction peaks; onset of menses, with lengthy, irregular cycles with gradual stabilization, a tendency for dysmenhorrea	Changing premenstrual symptoms within first three years
Young adulthood 18–30	Assuming responsibility for self; developing capacity for committed relationships; making career decisions; facing reproduction	Psycho-neuroendocrine apparatus stabilized; menses becomes predictable; cycles become regulated	Stabilization of the experience of PMS
Middle adulthood 30–45	Awareness of the "biological clock"; climbing the career ladder; appraisal of one's life situation in terms of stagnation and discontent; loss of youthful illusions	Regular cycles, with slow decline in length and frequency; increasing fluctuation in ovarian-hormone production; beginning atrophy of ova; infertility problems	Slow intensification of premenstrual symptoms, with more emotional and cognitive symptoms early and increased physical symptoms late

continued on next page

Table 5-1 *continued*

LIFE STAGE	PSYCHOLOGICAL DEVELOPMENT	OVARIAN DEVELOPMENT	PMS AND PERIMENOPAUSE
Late adulthood 45–65	Acceptance of one's potential; reassessment of life purpose and goals; increase in options; changing roles *vis-à-vis* children and parents; new self-image; facing mortality	Marked ovarian instability, with shorter time between cycles; menses become increasingly irregular; menstrual flow changes; slow cessation of menses; completion of atrophy of ova	Further intensification of premenstrual symptoms; perimenopause begins and ends; menopause begins and transitions into post-menopause
Maturity 65+	Development of wisdom; reassessment of what is important; acceptance of aging and mortality; "reaping the benefits" of age	Ovaries largely inactive; medical conditions become challenges	Postmenopausal

Infancy and early childhood. The infant slowly learns to differentiate "me" and "not me." From that beginning point psychological development proceeds rapidly; the child develops a sense of attachment and connects and bonds with others. This assists in creating a sense of safety and trust—or fear—depending on the quality of attachments. During childhood the person develops a sense of gender identity (as early as ages three to four), a significant period that focuses on gender-specific traits. This is a time of rapid learning. It is during this time that the child experiences the basis for her self-concept. During early childhood the ovaries are slowly and quietly maturing, and the pituitary functions are developing the ability to activate the ovaries later.

Late childhood. During this stage the young female must develop the ability to interact effectively with her environment, including developing the ability to complete tasks that she begins. Her set of personal values is largely in place by the end of this stage. She also must learn ways of creating satisfying relationships with peers. Most girls in this stage become more focused externally, in terms of pleasing and nurturing others. In this stage the pituitary gland begins to stimulate the ovaries to secrete estrogen, progesterone, and testosterone. Secondary sex characteristics result from this beginning, while the girl is growing in stature and muscle mass. The onset of menses occurs late in this stage or early in the next.

Puberty. The events in this stage are triggered by testosterone. The onset of puberty is often a subtle phenomenon, and the timing of it cannot be measured exactly as the onset of menses can, which occurs during this stage. The age of puberty has, however, been lowering for about 150 years, probably due to improving nutrition and medicine. Attention on the effects of puberty on younger and younger girls has not been explored adequately, and it is possible that its psychological and social implications may have become more important. During puberty the female's secondary sex characteristics begin to mature. The ovarian hormones stimulate the appearance of budding breasts (estrogen) and growth of pubic and axillary hair (androgens, from the adrenal gland and ovaries). A surge of testosterone during puberty causes heightened sensitivity in the nipples and genitals, along with increased sexual desire and arousal, increased muscle tone, and heightened energy. Estrogen and testosterone generate increased bone density, leading to a growth spurt. The female is now capable of reproduction and must face that reality. The onset of menses can be a source of both fear and pride. The young woman may be comparing herself to peers, and may become increasingly self-conscious about her changing physical characteristics. The experience of heightened erotic development during this stage, with its corresponding sexual desire and arousal, may cause the female to experience inner conflicts regarding the attraction and risks of sexual activity. The young woman has her first experiences of premenstrual symptoms during puberty.

Adolescence. During this stage the female is completing the development of a sense of identity, working out conflicts that relate to dependency and autonomy, and facing challenges regarding intimacy. During adolescence she also develops the ability to fall in love. Her menstrual cycles can be erratic. She can miss menses, and her cycles can be elongated. She may also have painful periods (dysmenhorrea). During adolescence premenstrual symptoms change, with more emotional ones emerging first. Water retention and other physical symptoms of PMS become more pronounced later in this stage.

> *Nina* is fourteen, and she is concerned about her weight and being liked by her peers. She began menses at age twelve. Prior to that she had a growth

spurt, and she became "pudgy." She has lost much of the weight, but she is still self-conscious. She says that her weight gain and rapid change in stature surprised and greatly concerned her at the time. During her first year after beginning menses her periods were highly irregular, sometimes every two to three weeks. During the past year her menstrual cycle has become longer and regular. She is beginning to ask questions about sex, and her father, who is her caretaker, seems reluctant to offer advice. He did not prepare her for what would happen as her body changed. She has been having painful periods, and she has been staying home from school as a result. She is beginning to notice some water retention and fatigue, and her father says that she seems to be more moody and difficult to live with.

This case shows changes that a female can experience from late childhood to early adolescence. At this developmental stage females often have few skills with which to deal with premenstrual and menstrual symptoms, interpersonal relationships, and self-affirmation. The challenge for parents is to develop the knowledge, courage, and skill to be resourceful to their daughters as they go through this stage.

Young adulthood. During this stage the young woman is probably at her peak in physical ability. She is exploring her budding adult identity and her place in the adult world. She is probably pursuing the aspirations of her youth. This is a time of rich satisfaction in sexual activity, love, family life, career advancement, and goal attainment. She must assume responsibility for herself, develop the capacity for committed relationships, learn fiscal restraint, and make career decisions. She has to achieve a balance between growing, learning, and achieving and the demands of her family, community, and society in general. She often has to determine whether and when she will conceive during this stage. The psycho-neuroendocrine system, which is an interaction of three key aspects of internal functioning, becomes stabilized. Her menstrual cycles become more regular and predictable. Her premenstrual symptoms form a clear pattern.

> *Megan,* twenty-six, is a computer programmer in a large high-tech company. She is ambitious, and she intends to "climb the ladder" in this organization. She is in a committed heterosexual relationship, planning on marrying within the next year. She wants to have children before age thirty, and she is concerned about juggling this with her career aspirations. She has been on oral contraceptives for the past few years, and she is having some predictable premenstrual symptoms. She experiences some moodiness, and she worries about that interfering with her work and her relationship. Her female friends are very supportive of her and each other, and she can talk freely with most of them about her career, relationship, and changes in her menstrual cycle. She and her boyfriend talk openly about her PMS, and together they strategize about how she should handle it.

This young woman has a healthy approach to managing her life and her physiological changes. Not every woman in this life stage handles change so well. If you are having difficulty, it is important to identify options to work through it.

Middle adulthood. Many women in this stage become acutely aware of their "biological clock" as they face decisions regarding reproduction. This is a time when women who have delayed conception until their late thirties to mid-forties experience fertility problems. During the thirties women in general report more emotional and cognitive premenstrual symptoms. This may account for the media's portrayal of PMS as a problem of the thirties. Toward the end of middle adulthood women complain increasingly about physical premenstrual symptoms, while they still report similar levels of emotional and cognitive difficulties. During middle adulthood women are often busy climbing the career ladder and juggling often conflicting demands of work and family life. This may lead to an appraisal of one's life situation in terms of stagnation and discontent. Many women are struggling with economic and emotional demands such as taking care of their parents, supporting their children's independence, marital discord, starting a new family, and organizational downsizing. During this time women often lose their youthful illusions. Aging becomes more apparent, and women can no longer think of themselves as "bulletproof," with increased awareness of physical vulnerability.

> *Peg* is physician, and she conducts clinical research on heart disease and has an active private practice. She is thirty-five, divorced, and childless. She says that she feels okay about not having children. Part of her daily routine includes jogging or swimming, but she eats irregularly at times since she is extremely busy. Her new domestic partner, Ellen, is a rising young attorney who is just as busy. Peg is having significant difficulty with PMS. She gets "mood jags," but she is more troubled by feeling down and quick-tempered so often. She has to be cautious about how she converses with both patients and coworkers since she often is impatient with them. She notices that she is having more joint aches and pains, particularly in her knees and lower back. This condition seems to worsen before her periods. She

gains three to four pounds just before her periods, and this bloating is interfering with her exercise routine.

This well-educated woman appears to be unaware that her ovarian hormones are having major effects on her well-being. Her neglect of her nutrition and her inattention to managing her stress may be exacerbating her condition. Her transition from a hetero-sexual marriage to a lesbian relationship is probably adding pressure on her coping skills.

> *Brenda* is forty-one and district sales manager for a chain of camera stores. She has three children by the last two of her three husbands. She has been attempting to balance childcare with holding down her job and pleasing her current husband. She has also been having an affair for the past year with one of her coworkers, meeting him once or twice a week for "quickies." She tends to drink heavily at parties, and she has begun to drink at home at night to unwind. She is having trouble dealing with her children, and she tends to lash out for small things during the time before her periods. Afterward, she feels remorseful, but the damage has been done. She engages in verbally abusive exchanges with her husband, and this has been escalating recently. She has become greatly concerned about how out of control she feels about her entire life situation, and she is blaming all of her difficulties on PMS.

This woman's consciousness about going through middle adulthood is decidedly low. She has little understanding of how her changing physiology is affecting her moods, relationships, and sense of self. Her coping strategies are clearly self-destructive, and this adds to the intensity of her life situation. Her mental and physical health are at risk.

Late adulthood. Women in this stage typically experience a slow decline in physical ability, with loss of reproductive capacity. Without treatment, they may also have an increased loss of bone mass and mineral content, slowing metabolism, changes in cholesterol levels (disposing them to cardiovascular disease), and skeletomuscular complications. During this stage women need to come to accept their potential as well as limitations. Often they engage in a reassessment of their life purpose and goals. Their roles may change significantly in relation to their children, grandchildren, and parents. They may begin a new committed relationship, enter a new family situation, and face many new options and challenges. Women often develop a new self-image as they age and begin to face mortality. During this life stage many women engage in what is called "generativity." That is, they attempt to pass on to the younger generation what they have learned. They become more giving, creative, responsible both for self and others, and more capable of sensual loving. This development can help avoid a sense of emptiness that women tend to experience during this time. There may be marked ovarian instability during this stage, slowly progressing into the cessation of ovarian functioning. Menses become increasingly irregular, with shorter time between cycles. Menstrual flow changes, either heavier or lighter, slowly moving to cessation of menses. There is further intensification of premenstrual symptoms, without treatment, through perimenopause until menopause begins. Postmenopause is the time when women no longer have periods for at least one year. At the end of this life stage most women are postmenopausal.

> *Josie* is forty-eight, married for twenty-five years to a successful entrepreneur. They have two children, who are both preparing to move away. One is in high school, and the other begins college in a few months. She has been a homemaker and very involved in

community and school activities. She is raising funds for an organization that is concerned with women's health. Painting has been her hobby for many years, and she has her work on display throughout her house. She is very depressed, and she feels that she is "in a black hole." She is questioning the meaning of her life. She says that she has never put herself first, always putting the needs of her family ahead of hers. She is panicky when she thinks at all about her future. She has little or no sexual desire these days. Two years ago hot flushes and vaginal dryness bothered her, and she began hormone replacement therapy. She has struggled with finding the proper types and doses. She is wondering whether her moods are related to her changing hormones.

This woman is typical of many who suffer from perimenopause while undergoing change within their sense of themselves and change within their families. Midlife crises are real for many women. Clearly the emotional impact of changes during this life stage influences your physiology and vice versa. Hormonal variations affect you psychologically, and this in turn affects your physical health.

Constance is fifty-three, and she was diagnosed as having insulin-dependent diabetes at age thirty-six. She suffers from some nerve damage in her feet, and she has lost some feeling in her fingers. Lately she has been undergoing laser treatments for diabetic retinopathy. She works as a technical writer for a software development firm, and her reputation at work is impeccable. She has been married to an architect for thirty years, and they have a grown daughter and two grandchildren. Her husband had heart-bypass surgery a few months ago, and she has been attempting to get him to change his lifestyle as a result. She has turned toward an alternative medicine approach to complement her insulin treatment. She used to have regular periods, but during the last two years her cycles have become sporadic. She is losing hair, and she is complaining of the appearance of hair on her chin. She has been having urinary "leaks" when she exerts herself, and she is concerned about embarrassing herself and others as a result. For the first time in her life she is having intense headaches and nausea. Her physician has recently diagnosed these as migraines. She has been experimenting with homeopathy and considering additional medical treatment. Her physician recommends estrogen and testosterone as part of her daily regime, but she is reluctant to become dependent on them. Since she has spent a lot of time reflecting on her immortality as a result of the complications of diabetes and her husband's health, she questions the wisdom of receiving more medical treatment.

This woman's situation exemplifies the complexity of decisions that women face in this life stage. Weighing options in light of your personal and medical history is imperative to making wise choices. Sometimes you get conflicting advice. Looking inwardly into what your life means can help when assessing and committing to a course of action.

Maturity. This is the stage that has been lengthened the most due to advances in medicine and lifestyle changes. During this stage medical conditions can become the challenge. Women who reach maturity often seem wiser, perhaps because they engage in reflection for long periods of time about circumstances, sifting out what is important from what is not. This can be a time when women can reap the benefits of long life, doing things they may have put off doing as younger women, including playing and spending time with friends. One developmental task in this stage is acceptance of mortality. Loss of loved ones can lead to feelings of aloneness, and women may need to develop new support systems for themselves as a result. Mature women's ovaries are largely inactive postmenopausally. Hormone replacement may be an essential part of managing the effects of the aging process. This stage can be very long, and the choices facing women in their older years can easily multiply rather than diminish.

Physical change and psychological development are interdependent. That is, they affect each other continuously. Ovarian and adrenal changes can bring about corresponding changes in our emotions and how we think. In turn, how we think can affect our physiological condition. These developments may not be linear, proceeding at a regular pace throughout our lives. Your ovaries may propel you into another life stage, or you may remain biologically young for longer than most women.

6

How Stress, Burnout, and Life Events Relate to Ovarian Change

Julie is a forty-two-year-old business owner whose company has tripled its sales during the past twelve months. She has recruited, trained, and supervised a growing work force. Although she has been single for ten years, she has recently fallen in love and is now living with a man who is about her age and has custody of his six-year-old son. She is attempting to "mother" his son, and she is enjoying it even though she is just learning how. Lately she has been losing interest in her business, and she has been spending more and more time with her new family. She reports that her work motivation, which is usually high, is low. This worries her intensely. She cannot seem to comprehend how she could feel so good in her personal life and so unproductive in her work.

Her premenstrual mood swings are more intense, ranging from anxiety to irritability. Her energy level has been markedly low just before her periods. She also reports that her thinking sometimes becomes slow and unreliable. She has trouble making business decisions that were easy for her earlier. She has stomach upsets, and she seems to have become allergic to foods that she once enjoyed. Her menstrual cycles are regular, and her menstrual flow has not changed appreciably in years.

Julie's life situation represents a number of dangers that busy women often face. Everyone's life has stresses and strains, but involving yourself in many endeavors that take time and energy can increase the chances that your premenstrual and perimenopausal symptoms will interfere with your well being. Stress is a normal part of daily living. Most people learn to expect it and develop ways of dealing with it so that it does not interfere with what they want to do. When stress becomes intolerable, however, it can have negative effects on your attitude, energy level, ovarian-hormone levels, and your behavior toward yourself and others.

Stress is the pressure you feel to respond to something in your environment that is pushing you. You are being stressed when you are required to react to demands, either internal or external, that force you to act. Sometimes the process is unconscious. You may be unaware that you are putting stress on yourself, and you may not notice the stress that your body is undergoing. As Walt Kelly's cartoon character Pogo said, "We have met the enemy, and they is us." You may be stressing yourself by establishing unrealistic expectations of yourself or others, and you may be living in such a way that your body is not being nourished adequately. You may feel that you must live up to others' standards, some of which may not fit with your sense of what you want to do. You may be continuing to live by the "no-no's" of your up-bringing, and as a result you may be experiencing guilt over mapping out your own way.

Burnout is a result of prolonged stress. You are "burned out" when your personal energy has become depleted to the point that you are unable to perform at the level of your former capability. The primary symptom of burnout is job-related stress. Having a lot of "unfinished business" and worrying about personal finances are other contributors to this serious condition. As we will discuss later in this chapter, researchers have isolated numerous factors that account for burnout.

Sometimes things happen and you are forced to respond. Research has focused on critical "life events," such as the death of a loved one, as they relate to your well-being and ability to cope. As we discuss later in this chapter, these occurrences can have serious effects on your *psyche* and *soma,* or your mental and physical health.

Stress, burnout, and life events interact with your physiological and psychological state at any given time. If you are premenstrual, stress, burnout, and significant life events may intensify your symptoms. Distinctions between stress, burnout, and life events are more apparent than real. In fact, life events generate stress, and if they continue, they can result in burnout. The hormonal fluctuations that you experience cyclically can both affect and be affected by the mix of stress, burnout, and life events that you face.

Figure 6-1 illustrates the processes that underlie stress and burnout. Your stress may be a combination of external pressure and internal conflict. If the stress is acute, you are likely to go into a "fight-flight" mode, that is, you almost automatically resist and defend yourself. After the stress has gone away, you then rebound, or bounce back to normal, without lasting emotional or physical effects. If the stress is chronic or existing for some time, it will probably lead to burnout if you do not take care of it.

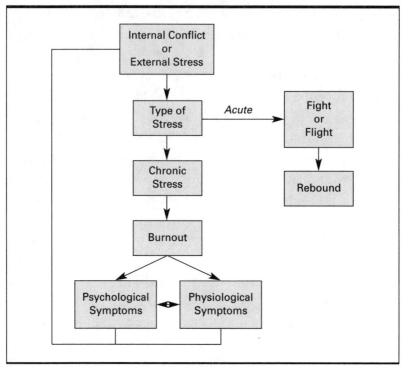

Figure 6-1

Prolonged stress, such as living with an abusive partner or working in an environment that places undue demands on you, can disrupt your biochemical balance. You may experience unusually altered adrenal-gland and thyroid activity, leading to such symptoms as headaches, high blood pressure, arteriosclerosis, colitis and other gastrointestinal distress, immune system disruptions, wide variations in blood glucose, lowered metabolism, and sleep disturbances. Psychological symptoms may become more chronic than episodic. For example, worrying about personal finances can become an obsession. Psychological symptoms that result from prolonged stress include depression, generalized anxiety, panic disorders, and compulsive disorders. The overall result of living under prolonged stress is burnout.

Your psychological and physiological symptoms of stress can exacerbate each other. Both can increase your internal and external stress. People may respond negatively toward your moods, and your physiological symptoms may make you accident prone, for example.

HORMONAL/BIOCHEMICAL CHANGE

Going through your menstrual cycle means that your brain and the rest of your body adjust to rising and falling levels of hormones that affect your emotions, mood, cognition, sexual desire and arousal, and behavior. This continuous change requires you to adapt to your particular cyclical patterns. Many women equate difficulties with PMS and perimenopause with stress. In fact, one common definition of PMS is *premenstrual stress*. The symptoms of these conditions, then, become stressors, to which women have to respond appropriately for relief and to maintain proper balance in their lives.

If you have an important event coming up and discover that during that time you will be in the luteal phase of your cycle, you may expect to be irritable, spacey, hypersensitive, and sleepless. If these are among your usual PMS symptoms, your concerns about their interfering with your project may actually increase their intensity. In other words, worrying about experiencing PMS may aggravate your symptoms. If you are perimenopausal, your inability to predict your symptoms, their intensity, and times of occurrence may cause you considerable distress. However, if you view this unpredictability as normal, you may not worry so much, and your symptoms may not be so intense.

With regard to biochemical changes and stress, the situation may be the classic "chicken and egg" question. Which causes the other? Studies have shown that women exposed to psychosocial stress had lowered levels of estrogen. On the other hand, studies have also found that having improper ovarian-hormone balance can cause stress reactions among women. This situation illustrates the delicate interrelatedness of mind and body. Declining levels of estrogen result in alterations in the neuro-transmitters (norepinephrine, serotonin, dopamine, and acetyl-choline) that regulate emotions, mood, cognition, sexual desire and arousal, and behavior. When you go through your cycle, hormonal changes evoke other body reactions that, consciously or not, you respond to. The symptoms of these changes can be stressful, especially if you perceive them as bothersome. And, living in a stressful environment can affect your body chemistry in ways that can accentuate your symptoms.

Situational, Psychological, Physiological, and Environmental Stressors

There are basically four categories of things that generate a stress reaction in humans. These clusters of stressors require the body to perceive, process, and respond to changes, both expected and unexpected.

Situational Stressors

This set includes sources of stress that are related to such things as work, home life, personal finances, relationships with others, your stage of development, and extended family conditions.

> *Pamela's* husband is a sales representative for an insurance company, and he spends considerable time with key clients after hours. She works as an administrative assistant for an accounting firm, and she has worked hard at leaving the work at the office so that she can devote her energy to her family in the evenings. Her children are ages eight and ten, and

she enjoys time with them. Lately her husband has been coming home late, sometimes bringing clients with him without letting her know beforehand. She is beginning to resent his lack of commitment to quality time with the family and his expectation that she will entertain his clients without notice. She is experiencing tension, anxiety, and hypersensitivity. For the first time she is having headaches and stomach distress.

Pamela's life situation illustrates the potential impact of situational stress. Prolonged exposure to such situations can lead to both emotional and physical changes, which, in turn, lower your ability to respond effectively. The stress is less of a problem than the situation itself. Being put into a living condition that is intolerable is, in a sense, victimizing Pamela. The solution is not in finding the proper medications and other treatments so much as in ameliorating the family situation itself. She needs to learn how to deal with her husband's changed behavior more effectively. We will discuss alternative approaches to such problem situations in Chapter 13.

Psychological Stressors

This category covers such phenomena as conflict within oneself or with others, difficult life decisions, illness of self or loved one, loss of loved one, significant disappointments, falling in love, falling out of love, and perceived failures or successes.

Mia is struggling with things she feels ambivalent about. She cannot decide whether to delay having children and whether to change to a job that she might enjoy more. Many of her friends are either pregnant or have recently given birth, and her parents want grandchildren. A coworker is making unwanted sexual advances toward her, and her boss is not taking the behavior seriously. She is feeling fearful that her biological clock is ticking fast, and this is interfering with her sleep. Also, she is tense much of the time, and her level of concentration at work has diminished.

This woman clearly has both internal and external stressors impinging on her. These two sets of pressure are interacting with each other to produce both psychological and physiological symptoms. Often psychotherapy can enable persons such as Mia to increase their ability to work their way through ambivalence in order to feel empowered to make decisions. We discuss psychotherapy treatment in Chapter 13.

Physiological Stressors

Included in this cluster are such things as medical conditions (either acute or chronic), changes in the level of hormones (thyroid, adrenal, or ovarian), and temporary conditions like gastrointestinal, bladder, allergic, and skelotomuscle distress.

> *Belle's* physician has recently diagnosed her physical condition as hyperthyroidism and irritable bowel syndrome. She has been jittery, anxious, and "hard to live with" for the past several months. Her seven-year-old child comes home from school with frequent colds and flu symptoms, and Belle feels that she cannot afford to catch these diseases. She is struggling with recurring bouts of diarrhea and is thinking that she may have become allergic to some foods. Her medical treatment has not stabilized, and she and her physician are searching for a proper solution.

This woman's stress is primarily physiological. It has become manifest in two serious medical conditions. Her physical state is acting as a stressor and is pressuring her to make major shifts in her lifestyle. The stress is probably negatively affecting her relationship with her family, and the frustration of not having a solution at hand may be further intensifying her illness conditions.

Environmental Stressors

These include such things as size of workspace, temperature in your environment, noise, safety, time pressure, performance pressure, and toxicity.

> *Toby* lives in an apartment complex, and she can hear much of what happens in her neighbors' units, particularly family conflicts. She works on an assembly line putting parts on computers. Her work climate is noisy, with an unpleasant odor and a great deal of time pressure. The line almost never stops, and she has to keep up so that the next person can do their part. She has lost hope of advancing herself and notices that her mood is down most of the time. She has little energy, and her interest in social activities has diminished. She rarely dates any more. She is beginning to become concerned that her life has lost meaning.

This woman is in a "pressure cooker." The stress of living and her working conditions have a decidedly negative effect on her sense of well-being. She may be moving toward a condition of anomie, in which she believes that nothing she could do would make a difference. Her major depression is leading her to alienate herself from people who might support her. Toby obviously needs to take charge of cleaning up her living and working conditions. She may be unable to do this on her own, and she may need professional treatment in the process of working her way into a condition of health. In Chapter 13 we discuss a number of alternate treatments that can assist women who suffer from environmental stress.

POSITIVE AND NEGATIVE STRESS

Not all stress is negative. We consciously choose to put ourselves under certain types of stress because they are enjoyable. For example, competing in sports, watching horror movies, participating in adventures—all these generate stress, but it is termed *eustress,* or positive stress. This type can leave you exhilarated and pleasantly tired. It may be necessary to have a portion of eustress in your life in order to avoid boredom and tedium. On the other hand, some stress has negative effects, and these conditions and events are termed *distress.* Distress takes energy away and leaves you with the need to cope, withstand, and draw upon your reserves.

Some stressors can motivate you, and others can *de*motivate you. For example, the stress of not having enough money can motivate you to get additional education or another job. Having a boss whom you do not respect can be demotivating, and you may begin to just "go through the motions" in your work. The same physiological symptoms can come up for you when you either fall in love or are frightened by a burglar. Your heart pounds, mind races, breathing quickens, muscles tense, and you may become temporarily speechless. These fight-flight reactions can be either positive or negative, depending on the situation. You may be motivated to either move toward the person or against him or her. The symptoms can be highly motivating—they move you toward action, in these cases either approach or avoidance and defense.

Sometimes, whether a stressor is positive or negative depends on how you perceive it. Some people seem predisposed to perceive almost everything that happens around them negatively. They are suspicious of the motives of others, and they think that everyone has a hidden agenda. These people are likely to perceive any situation in a negative light, and stress is almost always the result. Planning for a family vacation can cause you considerable stress if you see it as a burden. If you think about the planning as an opportunity for learning and maximizing your family's enjoyment, it can be a positive activity. Consider another situation. You are in a business meeting, and you receive feedback that your report needs major rewriting before it can be submitted to senior management. You can take this personally and become upset and defensive, even immobilized. On the other hand, you can take the feedback as helpful information for making improvements. The critical difference is in your interpretation. An exception is any life-threatening event, such as an earthquake. No matter how you perceive it while it is happening, you will feel stress, and your physiological state can even prevent you from doing the things you need to do in order to survive. You may be "frozen" and unable to react effectively. Clearing your perception involves both attaining proper perspective and communicating honestly with others. You may need to test the validity of assumptions that you may not even be aware that you are making.

A Matter of Degree

Not all stressors affect you equally, and any one stressor may not always impact you to the same degree. For example, you may experience more negative stress from having your significant other show up late for a date rather than from your car running out of gasoline. If, however, you need to drive quickly and have not budgeted time for possible car trouble, you may feel much more stress from that situation.

The degree of stress is largely a matter of how you perceive the situation. Some stressors are compelling, that is, you must respond to them right away. For example, you will need to get off the freeway and get some assistance when you have no fuel. The amount of stress that you experience in many cases is related to the sense you make out of the situation. Regarding the example of your significant other, you make yourself very upset because of the speculations that you make about that person's motivation, behavior, and the relationship.

HOW WE RESPOND TO STRESS

Stress is describable and self-diagnosing. The chief symptoms, or reactions, are listed in Table 6-1.

COGNITIVE	SOMATIC	BEHAVIORAL	EMOTIONAL
Slow thinking	Exhaustion, fatigue	Restlessness	Anxiety, panicky feelings
Impaired decision making	Appetite disturbances	Apathy	Depression, feeling sad
Difficulty in setting priorities	Sleeping difficulties	Nervousness	Irritability
Poor judgment	Loss of energy, headaches, gastrointestinal problems	Agitation, withdrawal	"Short fuse," overly excited

Table 6-1   Symptomatic reactions to stress

For healthy individuals, symptoms are usually followed by what is referred to as a "relaxation rebound period." When faced with a stressful situation, healthy people can bounce back quickly.

If an individual does not know how to handle such situations effectively, symptoms can become chronic.

Effectiveness in responding to stress can be jeopardized by a number of things that you can control. Figure 6-2 shows reaction to stress as a cycle of events.

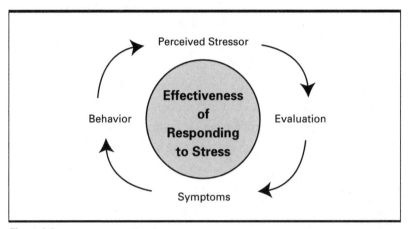

Figure 6-2

You perceive something as stressful, and then you evaluate both its degree of impact and your ability to handle it. You may reduce the resulting symptoms by affirming your competence in handling the situation, and you may be able to respond more quickly in an appropriate manner. If you appraise the situation to be more than you can deal with, your lack of confidence may actually heighten your symptoms. Your response to stress, then, is mediated by your sense of the whole situation and of your ability to respond effectively. If your behavior is inappropriate (throwing dishes, for example, or yelling at someone at work), the cycle repeats itself because you have increased the amount of stress in the situation rather than decreasing it. Over the long term, such behavior can seriously lessen your ability to respond effectively to stress. Vulnerability to stress comes from perceiving threats that may not exist or that should have less impact than you make them and the belief that you cannot change the situation.

The Costs of Doing It All

As we pointed out earlier, the net effect of experiencing prolonged stress is burnout. This condition is defined as a significantly lessened level of energy, such that you are unable to perform at a level that is normal for you. Your personal effectiveness is decreased. Research on this occurrence indicates that burnout is both predictable and preventable. Four factors contribute to "burning out": self-concept, habits, quality of relationships, and system stress. If your concept of yourself is negative, you are likely to be susceptible to burnout. If you engage in habitual behavior that is not responsive to the changing situations around you (and inside you), your behavior may not "pay off." Relationships with others should sustain and nurture you rather than deplete your energy. If you are locked in dysfunctional relationships, you are spending some of your energy coping with them. Following are the most common symptoms of burnout.

This list of symptoms is illustrative of the burnout syndrome. There are more than sixty symptoms that researchers have identified as directly related to this condition. Table 6-2 simply shows the most common ones. Respondents to the survey rated each symptom on a ten-point scale (ten is high), and these are the numbers of people who rated themselves as a 7+ on the symptoms. About one in three persons, on the average, reports having to deal with job-related stress to a high degree, for example. All these symptoms are modifiable through proactive behavior on your part. If you take charge of your own betterment, you can find ways to work your way through each of these burnout-inducing conditions. In Chapter 13 we spell out seventeen ways of avoiding burnout.

BURNOUT SYMPTOM	NUMBER OF PEOPLE WITH A HIGH DEGREE OF THE SYMPTOM
1. Job-related stress	1 out of 3
2. Unfinished business	1 out of 3
3. Worrying about personal finances	1 out of 3
4. Impatience	1 out of 3
5. Feeling tired	1 out of 4
6. Procrastinating	1 out of 4
7. Feeling tense	1 out of 4
8. Feeling unappreciated	1 out of 5
9. Avoiding confrontation	1 out of 5
10. Feeling pessimistic	1 out of 5

Source: Jones, J.E., and W.L. Bearley. *Managing Your Energy*. San Diego, Calif.: Performance & Human Development, 2000.

Table 6-2   Common symptoms of burnout

Having to cope with repetitive symptoms can be taxing and can result in having less energy for doing the things you want to do. Dealing with premenstrual or perimenopausal symptoms can be tiring, and you may lose your enthusiasm and motivation to engage in activities that you ordinarily enjoy or to accomplish goals in your work. Your symptoms or your inability to control them may lead you to conclude that you are an ineffective person. A negative view of self can be reinforced by how others around you respond to your behavior during those times when your symptoms are most pronounced. A number of premenstrual and perimenopausal symptoms include difficulties with other people.

The quality of your interactions with them may become diluted, and you may be left essentially alone. You are not receiving energy and encouragement, and you can be "running on your batteries."

STRESSFUL LIFE EVENTS

Things happen, and you inevitably react. Stressful life events are those occurrences that put pressure on you to respond, whether you want to or not. They are often out of your control or influence. Some are internal—they happen inside you. Others are external—they happen to you. Following are stressful life events:

- Divorce or marital separation
- Concluding that you are no longer desirable
- Adopting a child
- Death of a loved one
- Being laid off
- Changing residence
- Children leaving home
- Discovering that you have a serious illness
- Changing jobs or being transferred
- Having an automobile accident
- Having an unwanted pregnancy
- Having a baby
- Having a serious operation
- Getting a new boss
- Being promoted
- Problems with partner or child(ren)
- Financial setback
- Accidental injury

These events can cause different amounts of stress to different women at different times. For some women, for example, changing residences is joyful, while for others, traumatic. Losing a loved one may debilitate one person and leave another seemingly unaffected. Your reaction to these events expresses your personality, the ways you process information and respond to it, and how you relate to the expectations of others.

Facing stressful life events while having cyclical ovarian changes can be daunting. When you are having premenstrual and perimenopausal symptoms you have fewer resources with which to deal with the event. For example, you may have episodic hot flushes, followed by sleep disturbance. The next day you are having difficulty focusing your attention and functioning effectively at work. The phone on your desk rings, and you learn that your child has just been suspended from school for the first time. You already had enough to challenge you, and now this. If you usually have severe discomfort with your premenstrual symptoms, you may need all of your energy to remain reasonably effective. For example, you may be highly irritable, with frequent crying jags, and you may be constantly attempting to keep yourself in check while you interact with others. During dinner your partner expresses the intention of moving out. It may take all your resources to avoid becoming destructive.

As we point out in Chapter 13, handling stress effectively begins with monitoring the subtle changes within yourself, including ovarian-related cycles, emotional and cognitive fluctuations, and your behavior patterns in response to a changing environment. This seems like a lot to pay attention to, but you can learn how to increase your sensitivity to the factors that lead to burnout in order to prevent the condition.

The PMS Experience: A Matter of Degree

Every woman experiences the days just before her period differently. Researchers and health-care practitioners recognize premenstrual syndrome (PMS) as an array of emotional, cognitive, physical, and behavioral symptoms that occur cyclically during the premenstrual phase of the cycle and are followed by relief during menses. The two terms *premenstrual tension (PMT)* and *premenstrual syndrome (PMS)* have sometimes been used interchangeably. It is useful, however, to reserve the term *PMT* to refer to the emotional symptoms that occur premenstrually and *PMS* to refer to the complex of symptoms—both physical and psychological—that women experience in the days before their periods.

Premenstrual symptoms appear differently during the menstrual cycle. Some occur during the ovulatory phase, go away, and then recur premenstrually. Others begin during the ovulatory phase and remain until some time after menses.

The most common estimates are that 70 to 90 percent of the female population admit to experiencing premenstrual symptoms, with 10 to 40 percent reporting significant interference with daily functioning.

If you regularly experience some symptoms during the premenstrual phase of your cycle, you are probably suffering from some degree of PMS. This chapter includes the most common symptoms, research results on the severity of PMS, how to inventory your symptoms, and where PMS comes from.

TYPES AND CLUSTERS OF SYMPTOMS

Researchers have identified about 150 symptoms that women experience as distressful in the luteal phase of their cycles. We compiled a comprehensive list of these symptoms from an exhaustive survey of the available research and from a survey of clinical experts. Then we asked the same experts to isolate which were the most common. As a result we narrowed the list to eighty-eight symptoms, which we then studied on 878 women. We asked these women to rate each symptom on the level of discomfort they had with it premenstrually. We also asked these women to rate their overall level of PMS severity. An analysis of the eighty-eight symptoms put them into five clusters, listed below with illustrative symptoms. It is important to keep in mind that any premenstrual symptom can range from barely noticeable to incapacitating.

Cognitive-Attentional

This cluster refers to the degree to which PMS interferes with your thinking, attentiveness, concentration, ability to plan ahead, and ability to reason in stressful situations. Premenstrually you may have tendencies to misperceive and distort information, to be easily distracted, and to be forgetful. You may notice that during the days prior to your period you feel less focused and more easily distracted. You may "lose your place" while reading, writing, or even driving. Women who have severe PMS often become unable to make important decisions. If you have mild PMS, you may not even become cognizant of changes in your thinking patterns. This can contribute to a tendency to overreact to minor events. Women may need to be mindful of the potential influence that their other PMS symptoms can have on their thinking and concentration.

Heightened Emotionality

This cluster refers to the impact of PMS on emotional sensitivity. During the luteal phase of your cycle you may experience a number of emotional shifts, such as becoming irritable, feeling tense much of the time, and being depressed. Research indicates that aerobic exercise can significantly reduce the symptoms of many women with moderate to high premenstrual discomfort in this area. As we discuss in Chapter 13, psychotherapy has been found to reduce emotional distress associated with your menstrual cycle. You may want to reflect on what is working for you, and you may profitably accept that you have strengths to build on.

Physical Complaints

The symptoms in this cluster come from the physiological changes that occur naturally during your menstrual cycle. This cluster refers to the relative intensity of such symptoms as bodily aches and pains, lower backaches, cramping, clumsiness, leg pain, and other physical changes commonly associated with PMS. During the premenstrual phase you may expect to have general aches and pains, headaches, and lower backache, for example.

Women who suffer from physical complaints may be internalizing stressors. Psychotherapeutic intervention may focus on modifying this maladaptive style of coping with life situations. If you experience physical complaints premenstrually, you may keep a log of physical difficulties to analyze connections between your menstrual cycle and physical and emotional states. You may need to be examined by a physician, and you may benefit from learning relaxation and other stress management techniques, which we discuss in Chapter 13.

Sexual Behavior and Feelings

Your menstrual cycle is directly related to both sexual desire and arousal. This cluster refers to increases and decreases in interest in sex and actual changes in sexual activity that are often reported in conjunction with PMS. Many women report an increase in sexual desire but are often less sexually active during their luteal phases. In Chapter 11 we discuss how sex can get better during PMS and perimenopause, and in Chapter 13 we describe how you can improve your sexual relationships.

Eating Behavior/Water Retention

This cluster refers to increases in eating and drinking, water retention, bloating, and breast tenderness—all symptoms commonly associated with PMS. Weight gain, bingeing, and cravings for sweets and salty foods often are also part of the premenstrual experience. If you are suffering from these symptoms, you might consider consulting a nutritionist, talking with your physician to explore endocrine abnormalities, or seeking psychological intervention. You may need additional education regarding lifestyle changes, and you may also need to explore the possibility that you may have an eating disorder (e.g., compulsive eating, bulimia, and so on).

The entire list of eighty-eight symptoms appears later in this chapter.

PMS is a syndrome. This means that there are many ways of experiencing it. In general, any of the PMS symptoms that you experience throughout your menstrual cycle will show up to a greater degree premenstrually. Your particular set of symptoms and the amount of discomfort you experience premenstrually may change from puberty through menopause. Any of the symptoms that you experience most of the time, regardless of your cycle, can become exaggerated premenstrually. For example, if you are prone to depression, you may be more significantly depressed premenstrually. This pattern may occur with women who have such complaints as the following: general anxiousness, panic attacks, problems managing anger, or physical conditions such as aches and pains or chronic fatigue.

Do Women with Mild, Moderate, and Severe Discomfort Differ?

Women who classified themselves as having mild, moderate, or severe discomfort premenstrually differ significantly in a number of important characteristics. In our sample of 878 women 49 percent (1 out of 2 women) classified themselves as mild, 37 percent (about 1 out of 3) were moderate, and 14 percent (1 out of 7) were severe. "Mild" means that the woman's symptoms are not interfering with ordinary daily activities; "moderate" means that symptoms are getting in the way somewhat; and "severe" means that the woman's daily functioning is impaired during the premenstrual phase of her cycle.

> *Louise* hardly notices that her behavior changes during the days before her periods, but the people

around her certainly do. She becomes slightly grumpy and a bit irritable. She is aware when her breasts become tender about two to three days prior to her periods. She likes chocolate at any time, but during her premenstrual phase she has a more intense desire for it. Her two roommates have suggested that Louise may be experiencing premenstrual changes, since they notice a pattern to how her behavior shifts.

Dawn has premenstrual symptoms for about ten days in her menstrual cycle. She notices feeling down, being emotional, and crying easily, even while watching a comedy on television. She gets irritable and "short-fused" with members of her family. Her sleep cycle gets disrupted. She gets restless and has trouble sleeping though the night. She gains a few pounds each cycle, and she loses it shortly during the first one to two days during her periods. While she is experiencing PMS, her thinking sometimes becomes muddled, and she has difficulty concentrating and organizing her thoughts. She reports that about a day before her periods start she has intense headaches. Her partner complains that Dawn's moodiness is interfering with their relationship, saying, "You've got it," (implying PMS).

Lucia says that she has PMS symptoms for about two weeks before her periods. She gets edgy, feels overwhelmed, explodes at others, and becomes fearful that she may suffer from dire events. She is also afraid of losing control over her emotions. She has frequent thoughts of suicide during her premenstrual phase. She reports being forgetful, not being able to remember words and people's names, and she often cannot seem to focus on her work tasks effectively. She says that she cannot sleep on her stomach, which is usual for her, and she cannot stand having anyone or anything touch her breasts. Her abdominal bloating causes her extreme discomfort, and she gains five to eight pounds during the luteal phase of her cycle. She loses the weight within the first seventy-two hours after she gets her period. She is withdrawing from others, her career is suffering, and her marriage is under considerable stress.

These three classifications of women—mild, moderate, and severe—are similar in terms of the types of symptoms they experience. They are different, however, in the degree of discomfort they have. If you consider yourself "mild," for example, you may be feeling more tense than usual, while the "severe" woman may be extremely tense. Louise, Dawn, and Lucia illustrate how these three degrees of PMS get "lived out."

The three groups of women in our study differed with regard to when they experienced the onset of the symptoms and relief after menses. Women in the mild group had discomfort from one to three days prior to their periods; moderate women reported discomfort from four to seven days before their periods; and severe women indicated symptoms eight to fourteen days before menses. Mild women experienced relief within the first two days of their periods; severe women reported they did not experience relief until after two days into their periods; and moderate women were in between.

How you classify yourself (mild, moderate, or severe) is an important consideration. Think about how you usually function, that is, how you go about your daily activities most of the time. If your routines are largely unaffected during the premenstrual phase of your cycle, you are probably mild, or you may be having little or no PMS. If you notice that you are decidedly different during the luteal phase, you may be moderate. If your usual level of functioning is seriously impaired premenstrually, you are likely to be severe. Your severity level can also be affected by such factors as your medical condition, mental health, diet, exercise, and life stressors.

DO WOMEN OF DIFFERENT AGES HAVE DIFFERENT SYMPTOMS?

Some PMS symptoms begin as early as the onset of menses and increase in intensity as a woman ages. There are characteristic patterns of symptoms for women among different age groups. Our research found that younger women reported a higher degree of physical complaints, even though they experienced a wide array of other premenstrual symptoms. Women in their thirties reported more difficulty with cognitive functioning, emotionality, and change in sexual interest; and they also experienced a wide range of other premenstrual symptoms. Women in their thirties and early forties often seek treatment for their discomfort with PMS. During the fourth decade symptoms seem to intensify, particularly in the areas of emotional, cognitive, and physical complaints. Our research, however, found that women in their forties reported about the same level of distress in all groups of symptoms. As we pointed out in the first chapter, you can expect to experience premenstrual symptoms until you are postmenopausal. During the luteal phase of your cycle, you are likely to have at least mild discomfort because of fluctuating ovarian hormones.

Figure 7-1 Taking inventory of your PMS symptoms

Instructions: Rate each of the following symptoms according to the degree that you experience them during the week before your menstrual period. Use the following rating scale.

0 = *None.* I don't experience any difficulty with this.

1 = *Mild.* I have a mild amount of stress with this.

2 = *Moderate.* This symptom interferes with my personal effectiveness.

3 = *Severe.* This symptom seriously interferes with my functioning.

_____ 1. Fatigue

_____ 2. Breast fullness

_____ 3. Breast tenderness

_____ 4. Bloatedness

_____ 5. Headaches

_____ 6. Blurred vision

_____ 7. Increased thirst

_____ 8. Increased desire for alcohol

_____ 9. Increased intake of alcohol

_____ 10. Increased appetite

_____ 11. Increased sexual

interest

_____ 12. Decreased sexual

interest

_____ 13. Increased sexual behavior

_____ 14. Yelling and screaming easily

_____ 15. Being forgetful

_____ 16. Sleeping more

_____ 17. Disturbed sleep

patterns

_____ 18. Vivid dreams

_____ 19. Confusion

_____ 20. Being easily distracted

_____ 21. Increased use of

medications

_____ 22. Craving for sweets

_____ 23. Craving for salt

_____ 24. Pimples

_____ 25. Constipation

_____ 26. Night sweats

_____ 27. Oily skin

_____ 28. Lower backache

_____ 29. Cramping

_____ 30. Nausea

_____ 31. Lowered motor

coordination

continued on next page

Figure 7-1 *continued*

____ 32. General aches and pains	____ 53. Increase in arguments
____ 33. Weight gain	____ 54. Reckless driving
____ 34. Bursts of energy	____ 55. Binge eating
____ 35. Crying spells	____ 56. Putting myself down
____ 36. Irritability	____ 57. Feeling shameful for
____ 37. Overly sensitive	my thoughts and
____ 38. Outbursts of anger	behaviors
____ 39. Tension	____ 58. Procrastination
____ 40. Restlessness	____ 59. Being accident prone
____ 41. Thoughts of suicide	____ 60. Clumsiness
____ 42. Feeling inadequate	____ 61. Staying at home
____ 43. Wishing to be alone	____ 62. Avoiding social
____ 44. Not feeling like myself	activities
____ 45. Poor judgment	____ 63. Decreased efficiency
____ 46. Feeling lonely	____ 64. Mood swings
____ 47. Difficulty in getting	____ 65. Stomach distended
organized	____ 66. Increased urination
____ 48. Physical violence against	____ 67. Leg pain
person and/or property	____ 68. Feeling affectionate
____ 49. Lack of concern for the	____ 69. Avoiding intimacy
welfare of others	____ 70. Poor concentration
____ 50. Feeling indifferent	____ 71. Acting impulsively
____ 51. Feeling belligerent or	____ 72. Acting unpredictably
stubborn	____ 73. Feeling depressed
____ 52. Absence from work	____ 74. Feeling anxious

Figure 7-1 *continued*

____ 75. Lack of pleasure from ordinarily pleasurable activities	____ 82. Increased need to be cared for
	____ 83. Demanding
____ 76. Overreacting to normal occurrences	____ 84. Feeling helpless
	____ 85. Decreased exercise
____ 77. Thinking unusually slowly	____ 86. Difficulty thinking clearly
____ 78. Increased suspiciousness	
____ 79. Inability to plan ahead	____ 87. Difficulty making decisions
____ 80. Early morning waking	
____ 81. Needing reassurance	____ 88. Feeling the need to escape

ANALYZING YOUR PMS SYMPTOMS "PROFILE"

Remember that each woman has a unique pattern and level of intensity. There are no absolute standards. Look at your overall intensity level—the number of symptoms you rated 0, 1, 2, and 3. Would you classify yourself as mild, moderate, or severe overall?

Next, look for the symptoms that are giving you little or no discomfort (rated 0 or 1). You may have learned how to prevent these symptoms from interfering with your premenstrual functioning. There may be a cluster of these symptoms that stands out for you.

Look at the symptoms that you rated 2 or 3. These are the ones that describe your current particular sources of discomfort from PMS. Again, look for clusters of these symptoms, ones that seem related to each other.

Figure 7-2 PMS symptoms calendar

DAY OF THE CURRENT MONTH	POOR CONCENTRATION	OUTBURST OF ANGER	FEELING DEPRESSED	TENSION	HEADACHE	BLOATEDNESS	CRAVING FOR SWEETS	BREAST TENDERNESS
1.								
2.								
3.								
4.								
5.								
6.								
7.								
8.								
9.								
10.								

Keeping a PMS Calendar

You may construct a kind of calendar of your most common pre-menstrual symptoms. Figure 7-2 is an example of a PMS symptoms calendar. Complete it each day for two or three of your menstrual cycles, and analyze your patterns. Following is an example of such a form. Modify it according to your own experience.

Rate each of your most common symptoms each day on a 3-point scale.

1 = **Mild.** Does not interfere with normal activities.
2 = **Moderate.** Interferes with normal activities.
3 = **Severe.** Unable to perform normal activities.

Write a number in each cell for the day.

Calendaring your PMS symptoms can provide rich insight into when and how much discomfort you experience. You may also find this practice to be useful as you attempt to prevent or lessen the impact of these symptoms premenstrually.

In Chapter 13 we will discuss options for you to consider in coping with your PMS symptoms.

WHERE PMS COMES FROM

Since PMS shows up in both physical and psychological symptoms, its causes are many. The mind has a concept and an evaluation of self and a meaning system that interprets "reality" as it is perceived. The body has numerous physiological functions that change with age. As your mind and body interact, the result is a change in mood, behavior, or physical status. How the mind and body interact depends to some degree on the strength of your personal psychology. Think, for example, of twin women, with essentially the same physiology at birth. One develops a firm, positive sense of self, while the other engages in self-doubts and tends to view herself negatively. The meaning that they attach to their experiences will differ significantly, and this will affect their brain chemistries and resulting moods, behaviors, and physical statuses. The fact that they are conscious makes them active players in how their bodies react.

Your Psychology

Self-regard seems to be a critical factor in determining the level of your PMS symptoms. Other psychological factors that can influence your premenstrual experience include perception, attitude, processing information, and your ability to focus and attend to matters of importance. Women who are diagnosed with mood disorders, for example, tend to have exacerbated premenstrual symptoms that are related to the moods they are having difficulty with. If you tend to view yourself positively, tend not to distort reality (as most others would see it, including your emotional state), are optimistic, able to think clearly and methodically, and able to pay attention to what is important at the moment, your response to your PMS symptoms is likely to be manageable. You are able to see PMS symptoms from a larger perspective, not becoming caught up in the discomfort of the moment. Your beliefs about PMS can affect the level of discomfort you experience premenstrually. If you believe, for example, that women are unable to manage themselves well during the luteal phase, you are likely to make that prophecy come true for yourself.

Your Physiology

In terms of physiology, PMS is tied to neuroendocrine imbalance. As we pointed out in Chapter 1, your ovarian hormones (estrogen, progesterone, and testosterone) are affected by the chemistry of your brain and vice versa. In the brain neurotransmitters (serotonin, norepinephrine, dopamine, and acetylcholine) regulate your mood and behavior. They determine the balance among your ovarian hormones and the rate of change in their levels. In other words, the brain orders your body to manufacture these hormones and to keep them regulated. During the luteal phase of your cycle your estrogen (specifically, estradiol) level declines, progesterone dominates, and testosterone is lower than during other phases. This causes symptoms such as depression, crying episodes, sleep disturbances, anxiety, irritability, difficulty with concentration, and short-term memory disturbance. The decline of estrogen affects the neurotransmitters, resulting in mood and other changes. When estrogen is high, for example, there may an antidepressant and anti-anxiety effect. A low level can have the opposite effects. When progesterone is high, you may experience sedating and dampening effects; while a low level may have the opposite effect.

Your Diet

PMS is associated with dietary habits. The syndrome often includes craving for carbohydrate-rich (i.e., sweets) and salty foods. Eating a diet that emphasizes the consumption of complex carbohydrates and low levels of fat and protein has been found to lower several premenstrual symptoms, such as depression, tension, anger, confusion, lack of alertness, and fatigue. Serotonin plays a critical role in the regulation of appetite. Premenstrually serotonin may be lower, resulting in less control over your appetite. Your blood glucose (sugar) level may be lower premenstrually, causing you to experience such symptoms as increased food cravings, irritability, nervousness, and fatigue. Many women crave salty foods during the luteal phase of their cycles. Salt intake can intensify several PMS symptoms, such as bloatedness, breast tenderness, and weight gain. These symptoms are associated with water retention. Such stimulants as coffee, chocolate, black teas, etc. can intensify irritability, anxiety, tension, and depression—all common PMS symptoms. Research has found associations between PMS and deficiencies in several vitamins and minerals, especially vitamin B_6. See Chapter 13 for a discussion of food supplements.

Life Stressors

Research strongly suggests that stressful life events play a significant role in bringing on premenstrual symptoms. Our research focused on the relationship between PMS severity and symptoms. We found that women who reported severe problems with PMS had a higher incidence of arguments with their spouses, frequent illness, and problems with children than women with less PMS difficulty did. Researchers have also found that marital satisfaction is related to the intensity of PMS symptoms. During the follicular phase of the menstrual cycle heterosexual couples with and without PMS severity were about the same with regard to marital stress, but the ones with more intense PMS symptoms experienced more marital stress during the luteal phase. In other words, if you have severe difficulty with PMS, you are more likely to have problems at home and with your health premenstrually. Women who are employed outside their homes tend to have more intense PMS symptoms, and they report lessened productivity and more insecurity in the workplace. These findings clearly indicate that environmental stress plays an important role in your experience of PMS.

Prolonged stress can affect you both psychologically and physically. In general, stress adversely affects the neurotransmitters that in turn affect your ovarian functioning, leading to lowered estrogen. This can make it more difficult for you to cope with stress. Premenstrually, you have the added effect of "naturally" lowered estrogen, making it even more difficult to respond effectively to everyday stressors. In cases of severe stress, estrogen may become very low, ovulation ceases, and menses may stop. This can lead to amenorrhea, or a total absence of menses. In Chapter 13 we outline a number of suggestions for coping with PMS symptoms.

Your Cultural Background

Cultural factors may also affect your experience of PMS. Our research found a definite link between PMS severity and women's perceptions of their mothers', other family members', and friends' similar problems. However, research has failed to uncover any differences between women of different ethnic backgrounds with regard to PMS severity, prevalence, or symptom patterns. There is a clear lack of scientific knowledge regarding crosscultural samenesses and differences in the PMS experience.

Your Fitness

Physical fitness plays a significant role in PMS. Being physically fit usually means having cardiovascular health, sufficient strength to perform needed activities, the endurance to last through strenuous activities, and the flexibility to engage in normal body movement. Although there is no research that shows a perfect correlation between fitness and PMS, there does appear to be a link. There is a documented drop in athletic performance, for example, during the luteal phase. PMS can adversely affect several things that are important to performing well in physical activities. These include neuromuscular coordination, manual dexterity, and reaction time. If you are involved in activities that require normal levels of these functions, you are likely to be hampered during PMS.

Being physically fit is associated with elevated mood and enhanced positive feelings. If you are fit, you are also likely to have a higher level of self-regard, and that can help you cope with PMS symptoms effectively. The research on the relationship between exercise and PMS indicates that it decreases a number of premenstrual symptoms. Aerobic exercise that lasts thirty to forty minutes four to five times weekly has been found to effectively reduce PMS symptoms and can be as effective as a mild antidepressant medication in elevating mood.

If you are sedentary, that is, you do not regularly exercise, you can gain significant PMS symptom relief from even moderate forms of aerobic exercise, such as walking, biking, and swimming.

PMS is a life-engrossing condition for some women. For others, it is little more than a nuisance. The syndrome shows up in myriad symptoms, not all of which are experienced by every woman. Knowing your profile makes it easier for you to make choices about decreasing the severity of your symptoms, relating to others while you are premenstrual, and strengthening yourself in the process.

8

perimenopause: The Transitional Years

following are stories of six women who are in the developmental stage of perimenopause in which their ovaries are changing in unpredictable ways. They show different degrees of discomfort in living through this transition.

> *Lauren* is forty-eight. She still has two children living at home, aged ten and sixteen. She also has a son in his freshman year at college. Her marriage is stable. She has a master's degree in nursing, and she works as a clinical specialist in a hospital. She has been experiencing forgetfulness at times, and she "laughs it off." Coworkers tease her about being a bit moody during certain times of the month. Her periods have become irregular, and she cannot predict how heavy or light her menstrual flow will be.

Molly is fifty, and she has recently become a grand-mother. She manages a restaurant, and her career has been successful so far. She divorced three years ago, and she would like to marry again. She misses having a companion, but she does little or nothing to meet anyone satisfactory to her. She spends a lot of time alone at home, and she spends whatever social time she has with her daughter, son-in-law, and their new baby. She complains of having hot flushes at night, and this is interrupting her sleep patterns. She sometimes feels panicky during the day, for no apparent reason. She breaks out in a sweat during the day, regardless of the temperature in the place where she is. She says that she is often spacey: "I'm missing a beat on small things." She sometimes tends to blow a fuse when people ask her questions. Molly has begun consulting with a nutritionist and an acupuncturist in an effort to work out "natural" remedies for her symptoms. She is considering seeing a reproductive endocrinologist for assistance in managing her ovarian hormones.

Eva is fifty-one, single, and childless. She has lived with the same man for the past four years. She comes from a large, close family in which she is viewed as the main caretaker since the death of her parents. She works as a librarian, and she resists learning about computer systems, which seem to be engulfing her profession. Her supervisor is pressuring her to take courses, but she does not see the need. She suffers from fibromyalgia, and she is often so sore and stiff with so much joint pain in the morning that she feels almost unable to get up and get ready for work. She says that she does not remember not feeling depressed, but lately, she says that the depression has become more intense, and she is losing interest in the joys of life. Doing anything is an effort for Eva. Her relationship, although familiar, is not fulfilling, and she and her partner have silently agreed to withdraw from each other while continuing to live together. She complains of heart palpitations, and her urinary continence has become unpredictable. She has hot flushes frequently. She is on an antidepressant treatment, and she tends to take it more frequently than prescribed. Her consumption of alcohol has increased, which she uses to try to calm herself, but it is making her more depressed. Eva has discussed her symptoms with her physician, and the doctor has recommended that she begin hormone replacement therapy. She reports that she is afraid of the possible side effects.

Darla is forty-nine, living with the same man for six years. She works as a medical research technician. She has no children, and she enjoys sharing outdoor activities with her partner. She reports having had hot flushes about a year ago, but they have stopped. Her present symptoms are feeling depressed, with crying jags coming on without warning. Her thoughts seem more scattered, and she is often unable to find the words to describe what is going on around and inside her. Her energy is so low at times that the fatigue is overwhelming. She wants to nap during the middle of the day, regardless of the demands of her work. Until recently she has never had a weight problem, but recently she notices that she gains weight easily. For the first time she feels the need to be mindful of her diet. She is having vaginal dryness, and her libido is much lower than normal for her. This change is putting stress on her relationship with her partner, since he wants to engage in sex more often than she does. Darla, with the advice of her internist and a reproductive endocrinologist, has recently begun a regimen of estrogen and testosterone therapy. Her doctors plan to introduce progesterone as soon as she is stabilized on the other two supplements.

Lyn is forty-five, recently separated (at her own initiation) after twenty years of marriage. She has become attracted to someone else. Her two children, aged ten and fifteen, are living with her. She works as a paralegal, and her work situation contains considerable time pressure. She has had a history of asthma, and her physician has urged her to find ways of managing her stress more effectively. She is having generalized anxiety, with chronic worrying and irritability. She reports that she overreacts to her children's behavior and worries about becoming abusive with them. She recently rammed a fist through a wall at home. She describes herself as becoming verbally "unglued," yelling and screaming easily and unpredictably at home. She has frequent hot flushes, with a prickly sensation in the upper part of her body. She complains of feeling hotness and panicky. She says, "I'm just not thinking straight. It is affecting how I am functioning in my job, and I have been absent from work more lately. People are starting to notice." Lyn has begun hormone replacement and psychotherapy treatment in an effort to gain control of herself.

Brittany is forty-seven, a pharmacist in a hospital. She has a daughter, twenty-three, in graduate school. She was married for thirteen years, and she is currently in a live-in relationship with a female partner. All that she has noticed about her menstrual cycle is a very heavy flow during the past two months. This has been a surprise, since she had not had periods for about three months prior to the past two. She thought that she was done. She reports that when she was in her early forties she experienced moodiness premenstrually, but that slowly went away, and she does not remember any moodiness during the past year. Her skin has become drier and her hair is falling out more quickly than ever. Brittany has consulted with her gynecologist about her symptoms, and she has begun taking estrogen and progesterone supplements.

These women are experiencing "the change," the developmental phase that leads to the cessation of menses. They are having many of the symptoms associated with perimenopause, during middle and late adulthood. These cases illustrate how differently women go through this transition. Some, like Lauren and Brittany, have relatively mild symptoms. Others, like Molly and Darla, have moderate levels of symptoms. Finally, women like Lyn and Eva experience severe difficulty with perimenopausal symptoms. Regardless of the degree to which perimenopausal symptoms impact them, these six women are taking positive steps to improve their situations. As we discuss in Chapter 13, these women are using a variety of therapies to treat their symptoms.

WHAT IS PERIMENOPAUSE?

Perimenopause is the interval between regular ovarian menstrual cycles and cessation of ovarian function. Here are the most common characteristics of this transitional experience:

- Varying hormonal changes
- Slow, progressive, orderly change in symptoms
- Usually occurs during a woman's forties or fifties
- Irregular cycles
- Changes in menstrual flow, either increased or decreased
- Unpredictable fertility
- Intensification of premenstrual symptoms

Many people confuse the terms *menopause* and *perimenopause*. Technically, menopause is the cessation of menses, or your periods, and it is clinically defined as a lack of periods for at least one year and a significant decline in ovarian functioning. Perimenopause is the transition from regular to no menstrual cycles. This phase may occur quickly, but some women go though perimenopause for a number of years.

No two women go through perimenopause in the same manner. The beginning of the phase is related to ovarian age, which we discussed in Chapter 2. During perimenopause the ovaries become unstable, resulting in fluctuating hormone production and declining levels. This development leads to new and enhanced premenstrual and menstrual symptoms. Most women go through perimenopause during their forties.

Not all women experience difficulty going through perimenopause. Like PMS, it is a matter of degree. Your types and patterns of symptoms are unique to you, and you may or may not be bothered by them. They may cause you discomfort for some time and then change in their level of impact on your daily functioning. The challenge is to become aware of subtle and obvious symptoms and to find ways of living your life while dealing with them. Some women have mild symptoms, with little or no interference with normal activities. Others have moderate symptoms, with noticeable interference with day-to-day life situations. Women less fortunate experience perimenopausal symptoms to a severe degree, and this markedly disturbs their ability to carry out their tasks and enjoy living.

THE PHYSIOLOGY OF PERIMENOPAUSE

During perimenopause a number of biological changes occur. Ovarian follicles reach critically low levels. There is greater variability in the length of the menstrual cycle, typically decreasing, due to a reduction in the length of the follicular phase. The pituitary hormones, FSH and LH, have typically risen with age, in response to lower hormone levels produced by the ovaries. During perimenopause FSH increases faster than LH. The ratio between these two hormones gradually increases. If your menstrual cycles remain normal, these two hormones may also be normal or slightly elevated. If you are having long periods, you might expect an elevation of both or either FSH or LH, along with decreased estrogen (actually, estradiol) levels. At the end of long menstrual cycles, your estradiol level may be normal. If you are having shorter periods, you might expect normal or elevated FSH. You will probably have bursts of estradiol activity, rising and falling unpredictably.

All this indicates that if you are concerned about whether you are in perimenopause, you should take into account the variability of your cycle. Typically, health-care professionals diagnose perimenopause by measuring FSH, LH, estradiol, and sometimes testosterone levels. Ideally, all these should be measured. They expect women with ovarian instability to have elevated levels of FSH and LH, a low level of estradiol, and a low level of testosterone. A blood test, however, may not give you definitive information regarding whether you are perimenopausal. The hormone changes may be too subtle to be detected accurately by current methods. If you are in the early part of perimenopause, these measurements may be too crude, and laboratory tests may not reflect the symptoms you are experiencing. Diagnosis becomes more certain the closer you are to actual menopause. Your experience of perimenopause is unique, but it does have its own phases. Unfortunately, you may only be able to see these phases retrospectively. You may have a different set of physiological changes early in the perimenopause than you do during its middle, or as you approach menopause. The timing is also yours alone. The whole process can take anywhere from three to ten years. When you begin to experience menstrual cycle and flow changes, you can expect menopause to occur, on the average, about three years later.

New Symptoms

Premenstrual symptoms tend to intensify gradually during perimenopause. For example, if you have night sweats while experiencing PMS, you may notice that you are beginning to have heat waves during waking hours sporadically. One indicator, then, that you are perimenopausal is that you begin to have new body sensations and your PMS symptoms increase in severity. Here are the most common changes that you may notice, or become aware of as a result of tests, that tell you that you are perimenopausal:

- Shorter or longer menstrual cycles
- Change in menstrual flow
- Menstrual flow between cycles
- Periodic hot flushes
- Decrease in vaginal lubrication
- Increase in vaginal infections

- Increase in urinary urgency
- Increase in urinary-tract infections
- Change in skin texture and tone
- Change in bone-mineral content and strength
- Change in sexual desire and responsiveness
- Changeability of moods
- Increased anxiety, depression, and irritability
- Increased sensitivity to criticism
- Increased negative emotional responses to others
- Decreased energy
- Sleep disturbances
- Less facility in short-term memory
- Decreased ability to recall words and names
- Lessened ability to concentrate
- Cravings for sweets and alcohol
- Increased water retention (breast tenderness, abdominal bloating)
- Periodic heart palpitations

It is important to remember that not all women experience this entire list and that women vary widely in the degree of discomfort they have with the symptoms that emerge during perimenopause. Your awareness of and readiness to report your unique set of symptoms are critical to diagnosing perimenopause. You need to track your own symptoms. You may choose to keep a diary of your perimenopausal symptoms in order to determine the patterns of changes that you are going through.

THE WOMAN'S EXPERIENCE
DURING PERIMENOPAUSE

Here are typical things that women say during this transitional phase of their lives.

I wake up hot and sweaty.

I'm not sleeping well.

I rant and rave, and this is not like me.

I often feel tensed out and panicky for no reason.

My heart feels like it is jumping out of my chest.

For the first time I'm having migraines.

I urinate frequently, and I don't feel that I have as much control over my bladder as I used to.

My joints are sore and painful, and this is something new to me.

I just don't have the interest in sex that I used to.

I seem to be gaining weight in places I never had trouble with before.

I forget people's names, even friends'.

I lost my way driving. Often I feel disoriented.

I get overly emotional, and I can't control myself.

I can't plan around my periods, since they are so unpredictable.

Sometimes my heart flutters and pounds, without any reason I'm aware of.

Sometimes sex is painful because I'm not lubricated enough.

These women's complaints come directly from physiological changes and hormonal and psychological responses to these changes. Observing your own changes is important when managing perimenopause and deciding on treatments for your symptoms. Later in this chapter we will show you how to construct a record-keeping system for your symptoms.

Medical Conditions Tend to Flare or Become Exacerbated

If you have a chronic medical condition, it is likely to be more worrisome during perimenopause. The fluctuation of your ovarian hormones and associated physiological changes tends to make your entire system less stable. Here are some conditions that can become exacerbated by the rapid hormonal fluctuations that characterize perimenopause:

Migraine headaches. Women experience these twice as often as men. They tend to occur when the young woman has her first period, within two days of menses, during pregnancy, and postmenopausally. Migraines seem to be triggered by either a drop or intensification of estradiol levels. Changes in testosterone level may also cause them. Clearly there is a link between the onset of migraines and ovarian-hormone fluctuations, but it is important to bear in mind that other things—weather, stress, food allergies, withdrawal from pain medications, etc.—might also trigger them.

Fibromyalgia/chronic pain. This is persistent pain that affects muscles, tendons, and ligaments. You might feel stiff and sore, especially in the morning, and you may have pain in the neck, trunk, and hips, as well as numbness, lower energy, and fatigue. The pain may be accompanied by changes in your mood and cognitive ability. The symptoms appear as your ovarian hormone levels change or decrease, as they do in perimenopause. About 80 percent of fibromyalgia patients are female, and they typically begin to have symptoms between ages thirty and fifty. The hormonal changes that women experience during perimenopause undoubtedly contribute to this condition.

Vaginal, urinary, and bladder changes. When estrogen levels decline, the lining of the smooth tissues of the vagina, urethra, and bladder lose both tone and elasticity. Urinary frequency and incontinence (difficulty in control) begin to appear as bothersome and embarrassing symptoms during the years preceding and following the menopause. You may begin to experience urinary "leaks" (affecting about 25 million women and about 40 percent of women between ages forty-five and sixty-five in the United States), vaginal dryness, itching and burning, painful penetration, and recurrent vaginal and urinary tract infections. Other factors can cause these symptoms, but it is clear that they are more pronounced during perimenopause, when hormonal fluctuations are more unstable.

Cardiovascular changes. Lowered estrogen levels lead to an increased risk of heart disease. During the ages of forty to sixty-five your risk of having cardiovascular disease is eight times higher than having reproductive cancer (breast, uterine, ovarian, vaginal, or cervical). Women with declining ovarian functioning have an increased risk of coronary artery disease. During perimenopause your ovarian-hormone levels change, and this jeopardizes several important protective mechanisms in your cardiovascular system. Estradiol normally helps to regulate your cholesterol by increasing HDL and decreasing LDL. This, in turn, prevents plaque and clot formation, improves circulation, and probably indirectly regulates blood pressure. Estradiol acts as an antioxidant, which can improve your immune system. Progesterone can counteract the beneficial effects of estradiol, and testosterone can have adverse effects on blood pressure and cholesterol. It is important to ensure that hormone replacement therapy includes proper dosages and careful monitoring of the cardiovascular system.

Weight gain. With changing ovarian-hormone levels there are changes in body composition, fat distribution, and metabolic rate. This can result in loss of muscle mass and strength and an increase in girth, even with a lower caloric intake. How physically active or sedentary you are can be a powerful mediator in determining whether you gain weight during perimenopause. Leading an active life and restricting food intake can, of course, minimize the weight gain.

Chronic fatigue. About three out of five people who complain of chronic fatigue are women, and their average age is about forty-one. The symptoms include low energy, a feeling of tiredness, lethargy, generalized muscle weakness and discomfort, mood changes, cognitive difficulties, depression, headaches, and painful lymph nodes. Many of these symptoms are similar to those brought on by declining ovarian functioning that characterizes perimenopause.

Gastrointestinal difficulties. These can worsen during perimenopause. Some women report varying symptoms from constipation to loose stools with the onset of menses. It is also common for women to complain of bloating, abdominal gas, and changes in bowel habits when their hormone levels change.

Asthma. Women report increased difficulties with this condition during perimenopause. If you have suffered from asthma premenstrually as a younger woman, you may discover that the condition is exacerbated during menopause.

Osteoporosis and skeletal change. Although this condition is thought of as a disease of old age, it can affect women at any age after puberty. Bone mass and density are at their peak levels between ages twenty-five and thirty and gradually decline thereafter. The condition is caused primarily by a decline in estrogen levels, which occurs significantly during perimenopause. Osteoporosis is also known as the "silent disease" because these changes may be occurring for years before you become aware of symptoms. Osteoporosis is characterized by decreases in bone mass and density. A woman loses bone density and strength during this phase of development, and it is probably caused by changes in ovarian functioning. There is also an increase in periodontal disease during perimenopause. You may need to ask your physician to be sensitive to these changes as you approach menopause. Some conditions can increase the risk of developing osteoporosis:

- Natural or surgically-induced perimenopause that comes before age forty-five
- A history of maternal osteoporosis in your family
- You come from a Caucasian or Asian heritage
- You have a small body frame
- You are of above-average height
- You are underweight
- You have an inactive lifestyle
- You smoke
- You use alcohol or caffeine excessively
- Your diet is low in calcium
- You exercise to an extreme degree

Additional Symptoms

Following are additional symptoms that can occur during perimenopause. They have probably not occurred in any intensity in previous life stages.

Palpitations (fluttering and pounding of the chest). These may occur when estrogen levels drop. The symptom can also signal both serious and mild heart problems, and it can accompany a panic disorder or food allergy. About 40 to 46 percent of women have palpitations during perimenopause. Most of these women experience the symptom due to hormonal fluctuations, but some probably have other medical conditions that need attention.

Hot flushes (or hot flashes). These are the most common complaints of women who are going through the perimenopause. Over 50 percent of women experience them, and of those about 80 percent have them for two years or less. Small percentages have them for over five years. Each woman experiences them differently in terms of patterns, frequency, intensity, and duration. Many factors may cause them. Women whose mothers had these vasomotor symptoms report significantly more hot flushes than women whose mothers did not. Women who had a significant degree of premenstrual symptoms and women who blush easily may expect more vasomotor symptoms during perimenopause. They can be triggered during marked hormonal fluctuations by such irritants as stress, alcohol, hot weather, hot drinks, and spicy foods. Hot flushes can disturb sleep patterns and can bring on feelings of temporary panic and generalized anxiety.

Skin changes. Skin changes are primarily a result of the loss of collagen, especially among women over forty. This is aggravated by a drop in ovarian hormones, specifically estrogen and testosterone. You may notice more drying, flaking, bruising, skin fragility, and wrinkles.

Abnormal uterine bleeding. This is defined as bleeding that occurs at intervals of twenty-one days or less and lasts for more than seven days. Abnormal ovarian functioning, particularly a decline in estrogen levels characteristic of perimenopause, usually causes the condition.

Sleep disturbances. Perimenopausal women frequently complain of insomnia, restlessness during sleep, and early-morning awakening. Changes in gonadal hormone levels can bring about these conditions, and during perimenopause the fluctuation of these hormones can cause significant disruptions in normal sleep patterns. When your estrogen level drops, your serotonin level drops, resulting in this complaint. Sleep disturbances may also be related to a decrease in estrogen levels, since estrogen has a sedative effect.

Changes in hair growth. Three conditions can arise during perimenopause: hirsuitism (unwanted hair growth), alopecia (loss of hair), and finer hair texture. These conditions appear to be related to improper levels of androgens. Since this hormone fluctuates during perimenopause, these hair-related symptoms become cause for concern.

It is important to pay particular attention to the possibility that those medical conditions present during menstrual cycle changes can worsen during perimenopause. You may also have new symptoms, so your health may need closer attention. Your health-care practitioners may need to consider your ovarian functioning as they evaluate your health and recommend treatments.

SOARING PMS: SYMPTOM CHANGES

As this and the preceding chapter show, PMS and perimenopause are part of living through the continuum of your life. The two phases of development differ, but they are more alike than different. You are, of course, the constant, so your overall pattern of symptoms and your lifestyle determine how much discomfort you experience as you age.

During perimenopause your typical premenstrual symptoms

can become significantly more intense. About 60 to 80 percent of women experience mild to moderate PMS symptoms during perimenopause. About 15 to 20 percent have marked luteal phase symptoms that can cause marriage and family difficulties.

Many women complain of midlife depression during perimenopause rather than after the menopause, because of declining and fluctuating hormonal levels and other midlife changes. The intensification can result from more negative attitudes and expectations. Although it is commonly believed that postmenopausal women have more depression, research indicates that the increase in depression comes during perimenopause.

Except for adolescence, the highest number of stressful life events comes during perimenopause. Women have to cope with many changes at home and work. Western culture places a high value on youth, and women become aware of negative associations with aging during perimenopause. The term *menopause* conjures up negative meanings for many women, so they tend to approach it with silent dread.

Increased PMS severity during perimenopause is related to socioeconomic and educational status, level of employment, cultural attitudes, negative expectations, meaningful relationships, and self-regard. Women with lower socioeconomic status report higher levels of discomfort with PMS symptoms. Women who expect perimenopause to be difficult may fulfill their own predictions. They may anticipate that perimenopause will be unmanageable, uncomfortable, embarrassing, and generally unpredictable. This then generates negative emotional responses and a lack of commitment to learn strategies for managing the experience. Being in a supportive, intimate relationship can help you to cope with the major life events that occur during perimenopause. Women with low self-esteem, who engage in self-doubt, and feel less empowered are more vulnerable to increased severity of PMS symptoms during perimenopause. If, on the other hand, you hold yourself in high esteem and feel influential over the events of your life, you can learn how to minimize the exacerbating effects of fluctuating hormones on your premenstrual symptoms.

Keeping a Perimenopause Calendar

You may construct a kind of "calendar" of your most common perimenopausal symptoms. Complete it each day for two or three of your menstrual cycles, and analyze your patterns. Figure 8-1 is an example of such a form. Modify it according to your own experience.

Rate each of your most common symptoms each day on a 3-point scale.

1 = **Mild.** Does not interfere with normal activities.
2 = **Moderate.** Interferes with normal activities.
3 = **Severe.** Unable to perform normal activities.

Write a number in each cell for the day.

Calendaring your perimenopausal symptoms can provide rich insight into *when* and *how much* discomfort you experience. You may also find this practice useful as you attempt to prevent or lessen the impact of these symptoms.

In Chapter 13 we will discuss options to consider in coping with your perimenopausal symptoms.

LIVING WITH UNPREDICTABILITY

There is a commonly held myth that women dread menopause. Since the term *menopause* is misleading, it is important to remember that postmenopause and perimenopause are not the same thing. Research shows that postmenopausal women do not consider the cessation of menses to have been a negative experience.

Figure 8-1   Perimenopause symptoms calendar

DAY OF THE CURRENT MONTH	MEMORY LAPSE	OUTBURST OF ANGER	FEELING DEPRESSED	TENSION	HEADACHE	HOT FLUSH	TROUBLE WITH SLEEP	DECREASED ENERGY
1.								
2.								
3.								
4.								
5.								
6.								
7.								
8.								
9.								
10.								

Perimenopausal women, however, have many changes to go through, and they may become concerned over the unpredictability of this phase of their lives.

Mental disorders tend to peak during ages thirty-five to forty-five, with the highest levels of depression among women during ages forty-five to sixty-six. About 40 percent of women have their first depressive episode during ages forty to sixty. During perimenopause, for about five years before menopause, the incidence of anxiety and depressive disorders increases, as compared to a low incidence among postmenopausal women.

During perimenopause, numerous changes impinge on women. The aging process confronts you with its inexorability. You will not be able to recapture your youthful look and feel. During perimenopause women are not as fertile as in their twenties, but they are still at risk for unplanned pregnancy since ovulation continues sporadically during the perimenopause. There is a 59 percent abortion rate among women over forty, second only to that among teenagers.

You will probably also begin to consider your own mortality, especially if you have parents whose aging becomes a concern or if they have passed on. If you have children, they may leave home during this time. Your career may peak during this phase of your life. You may become concerned about your intimate relationships, and you may spend time reevaluating your own worth as a person. Women often report that during perimenopause their overriding concern is "Where do I go from here?" This question takes on pressing importance during midlife.

Some women cope with perimenopausal changes better than others. Generally, women who are better "copers" and who have a strong sense of self ride easier with the ebb and flow of premenstrual changes. These include women with more education, full-time employment outside the home, intimate relationships, little family stress, and a positive outlook on midlife. Some women suffer through a "cycle of defeat." Their life experiences validate their negative expectations. If you tend to see perimenopause as unmanageable and loaded with fear and dread, you will probably be correct. If, on the other hand, you see this phase of you life as workable, and you affirm your ability to manage it, you may look back on this time positively. We will discuss ways of managing your perimenopausal experience in Chapter 13.

9

PMS, perimenopause, and Relationships

In the following scenarios the women show typical signs of PMS and perimenopause. All three situations also indicate that dealing with the symptoms of these two conditions can seriously affect your close relationships.

Scenario 1.

The telephone rings. A husband is calling a psychotherapist about his wife. "I think she's got it," he says, referring to PMS.

The therapist asks for more, and the man replies, "Well, every month she yells and screams and threatens to leave me. This has caused us to separate a month ago, and I am worried that she is not coming back."

The therapist inquires, "Does she recognize this pattern of behavior as a problem?"

He says, "No. She won't talk about it. She blames everything on me. When I bring up the subject, she starts calling me names. She tells me that I am crazy and can't possibly understand her. I don't know what to do."

"You called instead of her. Is she willing to talk with a therapist about the problems that you two are having?"

"Yeah, she would if it is seen as my problem and not hers. She would probably be too embarrassed to talk about her PMS."

Scenario 2.

After a physical examination the doctor is giving feedback to a female patient. The patient is forty-four years old and going through perimenopause.

She cries as she says, "I am not remembering things. I can't concentrate. I'm missing a beat on small things. I find myself getting irritable, and that's not like me. I have almost no energy these days. I can't predict my periods any more. My partner is complaining because I am just not feeling sexual. My desire is totally down. I can't even count on a good night's sleep. I wake up during the night, and I am sweating."

The doctor asks, "How long has this been going on?"

She replies, "For the past few months it's been getting worse. It seems like I can't get a handle on all this, and it's starting to really affect my career and my relationship."

The doctor asks, "Have you tracked your symptom changes?" She replies, "No, I just make notes in my datebook."

Scenario 3.

Two female friends are talking over coffee about their children.

One says, "My kids are driving me nuts. I get on them, and they fight me all the time these days."

Her friend replies, "Mine are really good, and they generally do what I say. But there are certain times when the least little thing will cause me to flare up at them. One of them left a jacket in the living room last night, and I started ranting and raving. It's not like me to do that."

The first woman comments, "My kids can cause me to blow up easily. I guess I'm just becoming some kind of grump."

Her friend adds, "I am beginning to think that my flare-ups are somehow related to my periods. I seem to be more difficult during those times of the month."

The first woman replies, "You may have something there. I think maybe I am more irritable these days, and that has been happening a lot during the past year or so. I get jumpy and tense easily. It makes me just want to stay home and not see anyone."

Then the second woman reflects, "I've been noticing that I gain weight and feel bloated just before I get my period. I think I gained 5 pounds during my last two cycles. It is true that I do crave chocolate then, but I have been trying to control myself."

Paying close attention to how your premenstrual and perimenopausal symptoms influence the way you relate to significant others in your life can produce large payoffs for you. You can learn how to communicate what is happening to you with people who need to know, and you can enroll others in helping you cope with your symptoms more effectively. A side benefit is that you can obtain more satisfaction in these relationships through clear communication and mutual support.

INTIMATE RELATIONSHIPS

Loving someone intimately usually involves both emotional and erotic attachment. Of course, you can be bonded closely with someone without being sexually attracted to him or her. The relationship could be intimate the other way, too; that is, you may be sexually involved without the emotional closeness commonly associated with the concept of love. A fulfilling intimate relationship involves a mutuality, meeting each other's needs and accepting and respecting each other's preferences and realities.

What does gender have to do with it? Women tend to express loving differently than men. Female "standards" for closeness focus more on the quality of the relationship rather than the frequency and intensity of sexual interaction. This is not to imply that sexual satisfaction is unimportant to women. It is just that the method of getting to intimacy is usually thought about differently by women. The relationship comes first, sex later, if at all. Women who are intimate with other women, whether as lesbians or bisexuals, bring a unique orientation to closeness. Research shows that the emphasis of their relationships is clearly on the quality of the emotional connection, with the sexual relationship as a secondary emphasis.

Love partners can determine much of your life fulfillment. Therefore it is vitally important to let intimate partners know all of the significant things about you—to share thoughts, feelings, preferences, and changes you are experiencing in mood, thinking patterns, sexual drive, and energy level. Your partner(s) should also know how your body is changing, including menstrual-cycle shifts and PMS or perimenopausal symptoms, and how all this affects your desire for closeness and intimacy. Later in this chapter we will discuss how to bring up such subjects and keep communications with your intimate other(s) alive.

FAMILY RELATIONS

How a family communicates about developmental changes, both physical and emotional, can shape lasting mindsets of young women and help define their self-concepts. A family's attitudes about menses, aging, beauty, sexuality, etc. will affect the young woman's responses to changes within her own body and her psyche. The meaning that she attaches to the onset of menses, for example, is often learned primarily within the family unit. Her response to the onset of menses can have highly significant effects on her sense of her femaleness, her gender identity, and her self-esteem. If her attitude is essentially negative, she may be subject to a more intense experience of PMS and perimenopause. Self-esteem tends to dip during puberty, especially among females. Research has shown that severity and type of PMS and peri-menopause symptoms are connected to how young women are prepared for the onset of menses. If they are led to view the onset of menses as a positive life experience ("Gee, now I am a woman at last"), they will have less difficulty with either PMS or peri-menopause later.

Families come in many forms. Some women have biological families, and others have adopted ones. Your family may consist only of your marriage relationship, or it may include children, parents, in-laws, and other relatives. It may center on your relationship with someone you are living with, and that may include children you have together or children from a previous relationship. You may be a single parent, and you may view your family as including the children's father. Nearly all combinations can be found in many neighborhoods. Regardless of the structure of your family, you need to be attentive to the role that your PMS or peri-menopause plays in how you relate to these people.

If you value what you receive from your family relations, you need to nurture them in order to continue to benefit. Otherwise you may discover that you have depleted others' patience with you. This may make it difficult for them to give you the support you need when encountering changing hormonal patterns. It is common for women to take out their frustrations on their families while somehow presenting themselves as "okay" at work. Some women experience embarrassment because they are being ineffective either at work, at home, or both. You may view yourself as not having control over important situations in your life. Moods tend to take over, and thinking fails you. Embarrassment, guilt, and remorse are heavy loads to carry, and they inevitably take their toll on family life. In addition, these toxic emotional reactions generate a sense of powerlessness that can cause you to devalue yourself. If you "take it out on the family," there is a good chance that you may need to develop skills for effective self-expression so that emotional reactions such as frustration do not "pile up." They can suddenly come out when you are more vulnerable, such as the premenstrual phase of your cycle, when intense hormonal fluctuations can occur.

Sharing your PMS and perimenopausal experiences with your family can be a growth activity for both you and the other members. Telling the other family members how your body is changing and how your PMS or perimenopausal symptoms are affecting you can lead to a new level of closeness within the family unit. You may need to educate other members about your physiology in the process. In many families talking about such subjects is taboo, so you may need to become assertive in opening the subject of what is happening to you as your hormones change.

FRIENDSHIPS

Making and having friends adds significant value to your life. Developing caring relationships with others outside the family means investing in them—sharing, spending time, engaging in joint activities, listening nonjudgmentally, exchanging favors, and so on. Being friends means being dependable and trustworthy. It means wanting what is good for the other person. The best friendships are unconditional, that is, you do not think, "I will care for you so long as you . . ." or "if you . . ." Friends do not keep score. There is no balance sheet. You know when a friendship is not working when you begin to wonder whether you can trust the other person with intimate information about yourself, when you seem to be the one who is giving and bending, when there is little joy in being with the person.

Ideally your partner is your best friend and you maintain quality friendships within your family. It is also important to develop a coterie of friends with whom you feel comfortable discussing what is going on with you. Holding onto information about yourself can accumulate into "unfinished business," and this carries tension with it. This accumulation of internal stress can result in a breakdown, either emotional or physical. Every significant change should be shared with one or more persons. Many people can act as confidants for you. You need to be able to confide in a set of close relations in order for them to be a resource for you as you go through life stages. As you age, you may find that friendships become more important. Young women often make friends with classmates whom they never see again after graduation. People respond to a need for belonging by continually joining groups. In time, people may drift away from each other and develop familial ties. If you have children, this often becomes the focus of your attention. As children move away or mature, you may tend to seek out other lasting friendships.

It is sometimes easier to talk with friends than with your family about physiological changes. Female friends often want to compare experiences in order to determine whether they are "normal." The exchange of information about treatments and strategies used to work through menstrual cycle–related conditions can become an important aspect of your interaction. Male friends sometimes need to be educated about your physiology and the effects of your ovarian changes, and they too can be a source of understanding and support from a different perspective. Confiding in a man about such matters can lead you to look at your behavior in a fresh way. This may also be a good way to "rehearse" how you talk with your intimate partner. The friend may even coach you on how to get your husband or male lover to understand and accept you while coping with PMS or perimenopause.

Work Relationships

Many women spend more time with their coworkers than with anyone else. Developing the ability to relate to them on a genuine basis can not only be personally satisfying but also actually improve work itself. Working with people you don't like or trust can be miserable, so it is important to think through how you relate to your colleagues. You are paid to relate to coworkers well enough to accomplish work tasks. You are not paid to fight and bicker. Conflict and disagreement can impair work productivity. If your PMS or perimenopause affects your moods, they will be expressed at work as well as elsewhere in your life. Your hormonal changes can also affect your work by impairing your ability to think clearly, make effective decisions, organize ideas, remember important information, and communicate fluently. Other women in your work environment may be having similar difficulties, and they may not be associating them with their menstrual cycles. Open discussions about such matters can enhance your communication with female coworkers and, at times, with male ones as well. Each situation is unique, and the best approach is to evaluate your subjective trust level before you decide whether and how to open the subject. Men at work may either feel reluctant to talk about your changing physiology and premenstrual symptoms or may exacerbate the situation by attributing everything you do to your menstrual cycle.

What you need at work is to have a climate of openness and interpersonal support. That does not mean that your team meetings need to turn into group therapy sessions. It does mean that you need the significant people to understand and accept what you are going through and to help you be effective in your work while you cope with ovarian change. This may entail taking some risks on your part. You can test whether your manager is open to knowing about your physical changes, you can confide in colleagues whom you trust, and you can seek assistance when you are less "together" cognitively. It may be easier to ask someone to assist you in organizing a presentation than to ask for emotional support.

YOUR MOTHER AND FATHER

Your attitudes about your gender identity and your self-esteem were shaped significantly during your childhood and under the influence of your parents. Your personal values were largely established by about ages ten to twelve, and you carry them throughout the rest of your life. There is a correlation between how early or late young women experience the onset of menses and when they go through menopause. In general, late menses is associated with early menopause. This pattern may be inherited. There is little research, however, regarding how this relates to the onset of perimenopause.

The available research evidence strongly suggests that your experience of PMS and perimenopause is in large part determined by your mother's experience and how she dealt with it. Whether or not she was open about her premenstrual discomfort can be a precursor to how you approach it—either with dread or as a natural female experience. Your recollection of your mother's premenstrual and perimenopausal symptoms is probably related to your own symptoms. If you think that your mother had significant discomfort premenstrually, you are likely to experience PMS or perimenopause in a similar manner. If you grew up in a "closed" family, in which such matters were rarely, if ever, discussed, you may have developed negative attitudes about having a menstrual cycle. This could cause you to have a greater variety and more intensity of premenstrual symptoms. Your "thinking makes it so."

In families where there is open communication between father and daughter(s), the daughter(s) reports less severe PMS and perimenopausal symptoms. Often young women will assume that their fathers already know about the onset of their menses. Those who have this perception of their fathers report significantly less PMS and perimenopausal symptoms. If the young woman sees both of her parents as knowing about her menarche, she is less likely to report significant discomfort premenstrually later, and she will tend to view menses more positively. Open disclosure concerning menstrual-related events in the young woman's life, then, is clearly associated with fewer and less intense premenstrual symptoms. Little is known about the long-term benefits of this open disclosure on women's experience with perimenopause decades later.

YOUR DAUGHTER(S)

Research indicates that young women get their information about the onset of menses primarily from their mothers, secondarily from school sources, and thirdly from their peers and older sisters.

If you have one or more young daughters, it is important that you help them to anticipate menarche as a positive life passage. Being unprepared can be terrifying for young women, across cultures.

You have the opportunity to contribute greatly by helping your daughter(s) prevent later premenstrual and perimenopausal difficulties by approaching womanhood as a positive state of being and becoming and that menarche is a sign of maturity. Interview studies have found that the later that women are given credible information about menarche the greater the likelihood that they will recall the experience as a negative event. Young women who see themselves as well-prepared report fewer premenstrual symptoms and less menstrual pain.

USING OTHERS TO HELP YOU MONITOR YOUR SYMPTOMS

Asking members of your family, significant other, coworkers, or friends to assist you in charting your premenstrual or perimenopausal symptoms can be valuable. You may not notice symptoms that others become aware of. You may also have a tendency to minimize the impact of your symptoms, while your associates may be the ones who are being impacted by them. You may be more irritable, for example, than you are letting yourself be aware of, and this may annoy or stress others in your environment. It can be helpful to solicit perceptions of others regarding your PMS and perimenopausal symptoms in order to "correct" your self-perceptions. Asking others for help also legitimizes their discussions about your PMS and perimenopausal experiences.

Your partner (or close friends) may keep a calendar of your premenstrual symptoms while you do the same independently. When you compare the two records, you may discover different types, severity levels, and patterns of symptoms. Remember that these are, in large part, subjective perceptions, but also remember the old adage, "Whatever appears to be is always more significant than what is." The two of you can learn from this practice by openly discussing differences in your perceptions of your experience. The exchange ideally leads to your mate's accepting your needs. Communicating at this level of candor and commitment can also lead to decisions regarding how you manage time, how you ensure quality in your relationship and life in general, and your overall well-being.

Figure 9-1 is a model of a calendar that your partner (or other close friends) can complete on your symptoms during a one month period. Modify the calendar to fit your needs and common symptoms.

Rate each of this person's most common PMS symptoms each day, using the following 3-point scale.

1 = **Mild.** Does not interfere with her normal activities.
2 = **Moderate.** Interferes with her normal activities.
3 = **Severe.** She is unable to perform normal activities.

Write a number in each cell for the day.

Figure 9-1 PMS symptoms calendar for partners

DAY OF THE CURRENT MONTH	REPORTS POOR CONCENTRATION	OUTBURST OF ANGER	APPEARING DEPRESSED	APPEARING TENSE	REPORTS HAVING HEADACHE	REPORTS BEING BLOATED	REPORTS CRAVING FOR SWEETS	REPORTS BREAST TENDERNESS
1.								
2.								
3.								
4.								
5.								
6.								
7.								
8.								
9.								
10.								

If you are perimenopausal, you may construct a kind of calendar of your most common symptoms in order to solicit feedback from your mate. Ask him or her to complete it each day for two or three of your menstrual cycles. Figure 9-2 is an example of such a form. Modify it according to your own experience.

Rate each of your most common symptoms each day on a 3-point scale.

 1 = **Mild.** Does not interfere with her normal activities.
 2 = **Moderate.** Interferes with her normal activities.
 3 = **Severe.** She is unable to perform normal activities.

Write a number in each cell for the day.

KEEPING THINGS CLEAR

Both PMS and perimenopause can produce stresses on your relationships, but nurturing your relationships will help ensure that people support you and that you are good for them as well. You need to become aware of what your communication tendencies are, particularly those that can be barriers to effective communication as ovarian change can intensify these behaviors. The place to begin is listening. This involves paying close attention to the messages that your body is sending to you as well as attending to others as nonjudgmentally as you can. You earn the right to be understood by understanding others on their terms. If your "inner talk," however, is noisy and unclear, you may want to start improving your relationships by first improving your relationship with yourself. How you think and feel about yourself sets the ceiling on what is possible in your relationships with others. If you do not trust yourself very much, for example, you may not be able to have trusting relationships with others. Concentrate on developing

Figure 9-2   Perimenopause symptoms calendar for partners

DAY OF THE CURRENT MONTH	SHOWS MEMORY LAPSE	SHOWS OUTBURST OF ANGER	REPORTS FEELING DEPRESSED	REPORTS FEELING TENSION	REPORTS FEELING HEADACHE	REPORTS HOT FLUSH	TROUBLE WITH SLEEP	REPORTS DECREASED ENERGY
1.								
2.								
3.								
4.								
5.								
6.								
7.								
8.								
9.								
10.								

self-confidence and self-liking. Claim your strengths and other positive qualities.

Keeping relationships with others clear means paying attention to their needs as well as yours. Your communications should be straightforward and supportive, in much the same way you want others to relate to you. Telling the truth, not withholding significant information, asking for suggestions about how you can improve with regard to them, and presenting yourself as a person who isn't in relationships can encourage others to relate to you satisfactorily. Your PMS and perimenopausal experiences are genuine parts of your life, and people who know and love you should share that part as well as relate to you "in role," as a wife, mother, sister, or friend.

When you know that you are likely to be experiencing PMS or perimenopausal symptoms that can seriously affect the quality of your communications with others, it is important to let people know beforehand, so that they do not jump to erroneous conclusions about you. Knowing your symptoms can make it easier for you to plan communications, monitor your own communication style, and enlist others in helping you keep your relationships clear. See Chapter 13 for ideas and strategies to keep your relationships with others clear.

10

Hysterectomy, oophorectomy, pms, and perimenopause

Many medical conditions can lead to the decision to undergo hysterectomy (surgical removal of the uterus) or oophorectomy (removal of the ovaries). The age at which this procedure is carried out varies widely.

Cece is thirty-nine. She is a personal trainer who works at a fitness center. She is single and has no children. Her physician has diagnosed her with a form of hyperplasia, in which the endometrial lining of the uterus becomes overgrown. For the past several months she has had heavy bleeding for three weeks out of each menstrual cycle, and her periods have become irregular. Premenstrually she experiences bloatedness, decreased energy, and restless sleep patterns. She is aware that going through hysterectomy will not affect her premenstrual symptoms. Her doctor is concerned that she could develop endometrial cancer. She has tried various hormone replacement regimens, but this has not controlled her dysfunctional bleeding. She looks forward positively to life after hysterectomy, when she can regain her quality of life.

Jocelyn is twenty-nine, married, with a four-year-old child. She works as a clothing designer. She has received treatment for two years for cervical dysplasia, and she has recently learned that this condition has become cancerous. Although she has not planned to have more children, the news that she can no long reproduce is distressing her greatly. She is talking with a therapist about her reactions to the anticipated loss of her uterus. She is ambivalent about the prospect of not having any more periods after the planned hysterectomy. She does not seem to understand how a hysterectomy will affect her, and she has many questions, such as, "Is this going to affect my ovaries?" and "Is this going to make sex different?" Her husband, who is very supportive, has wanted another child. Jocelyn reports that he is sad that she has to undergo the operation, and he, too, is concerned about their sex life afterward.

Andrea is thirty-one, divorced, with no children. She is in a committed relationship with a man. She has hoped to have children, but recent developments have forced her to change her thinking. Suffering for several years with endometriosis, she has had highly painful periods. The pain has slowly progressed into general pelvic pain, and this has become debilitating.

She has tried various treatments, including hormone-type supplements and a number of laparoscopic surgeries to attempt to ameliorate this condition. Her physician told her after her last laparoscopic surgery that her endometriosis is on the bowel. And he recommended that she have a hysterectomy and also consider an oophorectomy. Her PMS has been interfering with both her work and her personal life, and her doctor has told her, "If you have your ovaries removed, you won't have to worry about PMS any more." She is sad, with crying spells, and she questions the meaning of her life. These emotional conditions intensify premenstrually for her. On the one hand, Andrea looks at surgery as a way of obtaining relief, but on the other hand, she dislikes the thought of never having children. She is concerned that the surgery may have a negative effect on her current relationship. She has consulted with a number of health-care practitioners regarding the effects of removing her ovaries and has decided to leave them intact. She has been participating in an endometriosis support group, and the exchange among women of different ages and experiences has been helpful to her. Many report that hysterectomy gave them relief from pelvic pain.

Lupe is forty-eight, married for the second time, with three children. She works as an independent environmental consultant. She has been diagnosed with a uterine prolapse. The muscles have become weak, and her uterus is sagging down into her vagina. She has been experiencing perimenopausal symptoms, including periodic hot flushes, vaginal dryness, dry skin, mood swings, and a decrease in sexual drive. She is beginning to experience some urinary incontinence. She has been on estrogen progesterone, and testosterone replacement for the past year. This has given her some relief from her urinary incontinence, but it has not cured the condition completely. She has tried biofeedback muscle training to alleviate the condition. Her physician has told her that she could have surgery to re-suspend the uterus or she could choose to have it removed. Lupe is questioning how a hysterectomy might affect her moods, energy level, sexual functioning, weight, and skin. Although she has had all the children that she wants, she thinks of her uterus as connected to her femaleness. She is concerned that she will be less of a woman without it.

Annell is forty-two, single, with an active social life. She is a lesbian, and she works as a graphic design artist. During the past two years her uterine-fibroid condition has worsened. The fibroids have become enlarged, and she has significant dysfunctional bleeding. This condition is putting pressure on her bladder, and her urinary frequency has increased. She has always planned her activities around regular menstrual cycles, but lately this has become more difficult since her periods are less predictable. She wonders why she has to continue suffering from these changes, and her physician has recommended hysterectomy. She has not been bothered by premenstrual changes, but she has heard that after hysterectomy, a woman can go through menopause within a few years afterward. She wonders about how this might affect her. She has been consulting with a naturopath to determine whether there are alternatives to surgery.

Denise is fifty, with two grown children and one grandchild. She has been a widow for one year. Her husband was killed in an automobile accident. She is an interior decorator and is also a licensed real estate broker. Her history of PMS has been mild to moderate, but during the past two years she has been having more intense symptoms. Her husband's death seems to have magnified her depression and anxiety. She has sleep disturbances, and she reports more difficulties with memory and concentration. Her menstrual cycles have become irregular. She thinks that her abdominal bloating is premenstrual, but she has noticed that lately it has become chronic. She has attempted to lose weight, and she has been taking herbs to combat water retention. Her primary care physician has diagnosed her as perimenopausal, starting her on hormone replacement. Since her bloating has intensified, with gastrointestinal difficulties arising for the first time, Denise has consulted with her gynecologist for a second opinion. Her gynecologist has put her through tests that indicate that she may have ovarian cancer. She is inclined to undergo exploratory surgery in order to determine whether she has cancer, and she wants the surgeon to remove it if it exists. Her surgeon has explained to her that if the ovaries are cancerous, both the ovaries and the uterus will be removed. She is concerned about what her life will be like after surgery and is preoccupied with what it would mean not to have ovaries—more so than not to have a uterus. Denise has been working with a psychotherapist as a result of her husband's death, and she is exploring her concerns about her physical condition as well. She is wondering whether she will feel "neutered," whether she will age prematurely, and whether her depression and anxiety will continue or increase.

The dilemmas facing these six women illustrate the concerns surrounding hysterectomy and oophorectomy. These women face having parts of their bodies removed—parts that are intimately associated with their sexuality. All these cases show ambivalence about the surgery and a lack of understanding of the effects that hysterectomy and oophorectomy are likely to have. These women have many questions, and they vary in the degree to which they are actively seeking answers.

Women who face having their uteruses or ovaries removed anticipate the experience with almost a uniform sense of deep concern. Following are some common questions that they ask.

Will I feel different afterward?

Will I continue to enjoy sex?

Will I have to have hormone replacements?

Why doesn't my doctor ask me about my feelings about this?

Will my orgasms change?

Will it hurt a lot? For how long?

How long will it take to recuperate?

Will my partner notice anything different sexually? Will my thinking and emotions change afterwards?

Will the operation change my ability to do my physical activities?

Will it cure PMS?

Will I shrivel up and suddenly feel old?

Will I go into menopause?

Will the surgery take care of my perimenopausal symptoms?

If my ovaries are removed, how will I be different?

Will others think of me as 'used goods'?

Will my partner still be attracted to me?

Will I regain my energy?

If I have a hysterectomy, will I have to lose my ovaries, too?

Will losing my uterus affect my ovaries if I decide to keep them?

In addition to these concerns, hysterectomy and oophorectomy symbolize for some women the loss of a defining body part. It means having part of how they came into the world irreversibly altered. Some women associate having a uterus and ovaries with being young, and its loss with aging. Some associate hysterectomy and oophorectomy with their grandmothers, not with themselves. For women who are childless or who want to have additional children, there is the realization that they will not be able to carry one.

Women who experience a lot of pain, excessive bleeding, and general feelings of unhealthiness anticipate having a hysterectomy positively. The procedure not only can improve these conditions but also generate other positive outcomes. You are suddenly relieved of any fear of unwanted pregnancy, you no longer have the bother of periods, and you can plan your activities independent of menses. The procedure prevents the development of uterine and cervical cancer, and it can improve the overall quality of life.

If the ovaries are removed as part of the procedure, you can protect against ovarian cancer, but this practice is controversial. About 10 to 14 percent of ovarian cancers may be prevented through oophorectomy, but the decision to undergo the surgery needs to be done on a case-by-case basis. The present screening procedures for the early detection of ovarian cancer are unreliable and expensive. Screening indicators that are being studied include environmental factors, hormonal changes, and genetic predisposition. You are at a 30 to 50 percent risk of developing ovarian cancer if you have any of the following conditions within your family:

- Ovarian cancer
- Breast and ovarian cancer combined
- Cancers of the colon, prostate, lungs, or uterus

Other risk factors include frequent ovarian cysts, difficulties with the endocrine system, being overweight, having a diet high in animal fats, using tobacco products, and environmental pollutants.

Research into genetics is offering promise of predicting the development of ovarian cancer. Researchers are experimenting with ultrasound in detecting ovarian abnormality. While this procedure is more specific than pelvic examinations, it still does not provide enough information on which to base reliable judgments regarding the presence of cancer. One type of ultrasonography, transvaginal, offers the promise of detecting ovarian cancer in women who show no symptoms and for whom pelvic examinations fail to detect the condition. The Color Doppler technique studies the blood flow within the ovaries and can help distinguish normal and abnormal vessels, differentiating between malignant and benign tumors. Research into "biomarkers" may isolate specific indicators of ovarian cancer. The disease is usually detected in its later stages, but by then, the mortality rate is high.

Women anticipate having an oophorectomy with mixed feelings. For some women it represents freedom from having PMS and perimenopausal symptoms and prevention of disease. For others the thought of not having ovaries causes worry, fear, and concern over loss of the natural flow of hormones. Some women express concerns over whether they will be "de-sexed" and somehow lose their sense of femininity and attractiveness. They worry that not having ovaries will cause them to be moody, have low energy, and lose sexual functioning.

IS HYSTERECTOMY DIFFERENT FROM OOPHORECTOMY?

Women often confuse the terms *hysterectomy* and *oophorectomy*. Hysterectomy is the surgical removal of the uterus. It may be partial (the removal of the uterus and cervix) or complete (the removal of the uterus, cervix, and the fallopian tubes). A subtotal hysterectomy (supracervical) leaves the cervix in place. An oophorectomy is a surgical procedure that involves the removal of one or both ovaries (unilateral or bilateral salpingo-oophorectomy). One effect is that the woman no longer produces sufficient levels of the ovarian hormones. Ovariectomy is the removal of part of an ovary, to remove a cyst, for example. Physicians may contribute to this lack of clarity by using the term *hysterectomy* when both the uterus and one or both ovaries are surgically removed.

What necessitates a hysterectomy? The seven most common conditions that call for this operation are endometriosis, the presence of a tumor (either benign or cancerous), other forms of cancer (cervical, endometrial, or ovarian), a prolapsed uterus, intrauterine or other abnormal bleeding, life-threatening pelvic inflammatory disease, and pelvic pain (although the procedure may not relieve this). Endometriosis is a disease in which part of the lining of the uterus imbeds itself in parts of the pelvis, such as over the ovaries, inside the vagina, onto the bladder, and onto the bowels.

Hysterectomy procedures occur much more frequently in the United States than in any other industrialized nation. In the United States a woman is six times more likely to undergo a hysterectomy than in any other comparable place. Here are some facts about the incidence of hysterectomy and oophorectomy in the United States:

- There were 1.7 million hysterectomies between 1988 and 1990.
- Bilateral oophorectomy occurred in 50 percent of these surgeries.
- About 60 percent of hysterectomies were performed on women less than forty-five years of age.

The procedure has been used for over two thousand years, probably at first because of complications in childbearing. There are basically five types of this procedure:

- **Supracervical hysterectomy.** Removal of the fundus, or top, of the uterus only.
- **Partial hysterectomy.** Removal of the uterus and cervix.
- **Complete hysterectomy.** Removal of the entire uterus, including the body and the neck (the cervix) and fallopian tubes.
- **Radical hysterectomy.** Removal of the entire uterus, including the cervix, the top portion of the vagina (the vaginal cup), and much of the tissue that surrounds the cervix.
- **Hysterectomy and bilateral salpingo-oophorec-tomy.** Complete removal of the uterus, the ovaries, and the fallopian tubes.

Hysterectomy and oophorectomy can be carried out either vaginally or abdominally. When the procedure is carried out through an abdominal incision, two effects result, a scar about which you may become self-conscious and a stretching of the abdominal muscles, which can cause protruding of your abdomen for perhaps several months. Both the level of pain and general discomfort experienced after a hysterectomy and the time it takes to resume normal physical activity vary widely among women. Having the procedure done vaginally has advantages: recovery time is shorter and discomfort is minimized. Laparoscopically assisted vaginal hysterectomy allows for a greater percentage of these surgeries to have these two benefits.

Approximately 20 to 30 percent of women who undergo hysterectomies also have one or both of their ovaries removed. Oophorectomy is usually necessitated by the presence of benign or malignant tumors or by endometriosis. Oophorectomy causes an immediate cessation of ovarian hormones. This means that you no longer have periods, and your hormonal balance is disrupted because the major producers of estrogen, progesterone, and testosterone are removed. Medical researchers speculate that the ovaries produce other substances that have important functions, and their removal has some unforeseen consequences.

Deciding whether to undergo hysterectomy or oophorectomy is both complex and important. You may choose to get a second medical opinion before committing yourself to this procedure. In the process you may gain helpful information and insight into your medical condition. Psychological preparation for surgery, especially gynecological procedures, can assist you in alleviating fear and anxiety, and research shows that it also leads to a lessening of postoperative complications. Some health insurance companies encourage the practice of soliciting second opinions regarding such surgery since in some cases a procedure is not warranted.

AN ALTERNATIVE: MYOMECTOMY

This is a surgical procedure that removes diseased portions of the uterus, usually nonmalignant fibroid tumors or other growths, leaving the uterus intact. The operation takes place through the vagina or the abdomen. Reconstructing the uterus through this procedure can restore it to near-normal functioning. This means that normal uterine function—conception, glandular secretions from the endometrial lining, lubrication—can continue as before. While formerly carried out with younger women who were concerned about maintaining their reproductive capacity, this procedure is now used with middle-aged women who have delayed their childbearing and who want to preserve the blood supply to the ovaries to ensure normal hormone release.

A myomectomy maintains neuroendocrine control of the ovaries; that is, the uterus and ovaries interact properly so that the ovaries can continue to function as they did prior to surgery. The procedure requires a skillful surgeon. The uterus can be weaker after the procedure, and rupturing can occur. Postoperative problems may include bleeding, infection, and interference with bowel function. Deciding on this procedure is dependent on the size and position of the intrauterine growths. Fibroids recur in about 10 to 20 percent of women who undergo this procedure.

THE UTERUS AND OVARIES AS PSYCHOLOGICAL ORGANS

Women tend to consider the rhythm of their menstrual cycles as they plan daily activities. You may consider your cycle as you plan your sexual practices, reproduction goals, vacations, and physical activities.

Menses has symbolic meaning for women. It defines them

as feminine, and its onset is a cornerstone of development. Menses is connected to fertility, and women have strong feelings about being able to reproduce. Since this organ is weighted with emotional associations, having a uterus means that your body is still intact, that you are still young, and that your femininity has not been altered surgically.

One of the dangers of becoming hysterectomized and oophorectomized is that women can come to see themselves as less attractive as a sex partner and less desirable as a companion. A woman may feel that her "personhood" has changed, that she has to adapt to a new view of herself. Instead of attaching positive imagery to the experience, she may dwell on her loss or imagine her worst fantasy. She may remember tales about women who have lost their uteruses and ovaries and who had negative experiences as a result. A woman may, of course, take the opposite approach: reframing the experience to free herself of concerns about reproduction and an unhealthy physical condition.

Whether a woman actually wants children may not be as important as the ability to bear them. If you want more children than you already have and you want to bear them yourself, a uterus is a necessity. Since the uterus has no counterpart in the male physiology, you may think of it as a defining part of your femininity. Whether you realize it or not, the uterus is a rich contributor to your overall sense of well-being. It can influence the choices you make in the roles and relationships you deal with during your life.

The ovaries give you a "hormonal clock" that regulates both physical and emotional processes. In Chapter 2 we discuss how ovaries contribute to physical and emotional well-being. A major concern of women who are deciding about oophorectomy is whether hormonal supplements will adequately compensate for the natural source of estrogen, progesterone, and testosterone.

They also worry about how the removal of their ovaries will affect their day-to-day functioning.

Hysterectomy and oophorectomy are often thought of solely in terms of the removal of internal organs. Often there is little or no attention paid to the psychological effects of such procedures. Removal of what is distinctively female can represent powerful changes for women.

Differences After the Procedures

Strong emotions are often associated with the experience of hysterectomy and oophorectomy. First is the anxiety about hospitalization and surgery itself. These feelings are completely natural and predictable. Aside from this general concern are more specific fears: fear of surgical accidents, fear of the unknown, fear of anesthesia, fear of pain, fear of momentary and long-lasting effects, and fear of emotionally breaking down, showing excess emotion, or losing control. To some degree all of these concerns are normal. Discussing them with your health-care team can help reduce fears by increasing your understanding of the procedures and strengthening yourself in preparation for them. If your fears are paralyzing you, you may need to discuss them with a qualified psychotherapist (see Chapter 13).

The loss of a uterus loss represents the absence of a uniquely feminine organ, and this can affect how you think and feel about yourself as a woman. The disruption of the blood supply from the uterus to the ovaries alters their functioning and has an indirect effect on your brain chemistry (e.g., neurotransmitters and neuropeptides). This can result in changes in mood, energy level, and sex drive. If your cervix is removed, you may have a slight change in vaginal lubrication. Medical researchers speculate that the uterus produces chemical substances that interact with the ovaries, and removal of the uterus could have unknown effects.

Research has indicated that hysterectomy and oophorectomy increase the risk of developing osteoporosis, coronary artery disease, and genitourinary atrophy at a younger age. Women who have undergone hysterectomies without oophorectomy report the following physical symptoms afterward:

- Breast engorgement and pain
- Sleep disturbances
- Weight gain
- Gastrointestinal complaints
- Hair loss
- Premature graying
- Urinary incontinence

Women who have had hysterectomies and retained their ovaries have been found to have a more positive attitude toward the procedure and toward themselves, especially when the surgery gave them relief from dysfunctional bleeding or pelvic pain. About 15 percent experienced negative psychological consequences, such as sadness, emptiness, grief, and depressive thoughts. Their self-esteem was lower, and they were more negative about their femininity. Whether depression is an outcome of hysterectomy is dependent on your emotional stability, sexual identity, body image before surgery, and cultural background. Preparation for the experience should be an important part of your planning. You may decide to seek psychotherapeutic assistance in order to prepare yourself.

Hysterectomy can induce changes in your emotional experience. You may experience "postoperative blues," which involve continuous worrying about what your life will be like from that time on. You may even grieve the loss of a vital body part. You may be anxious about what this change will do to your general sense of well-being. Researchers have estimated that about 70 percent of women who become depressed after a hysterectomy need treatment within the first three years after the operation. Having preventive psychotherapy prior to the procedure minimizes this vulnerability.

There is no evidence that a hysterectomy will affect your ability to think and reason effectively. Your sexual desire and capacity for orgasm do not change. You may experience painful intercourse due to temporary shrinkage of the vagina, and you may also be bothered by less vaginal space if your cervix is removed. But research indicates that within about four months, about 90 percent of hysterectomized women are fully functional with regard to sexual intercourse. (There could be an indirect effect on sexual desire, arousal, and orgasm, in response to the lowered blood supply to the ovaries. We will discuss this in Chapter 11.)

Removal of the uterus and ovaries is a potentially life-changing experience. It can bring about changes in how you think about yourself; it can evoke significant feelings; and it can be a springboard to reaffirming yourself as a woman, with a new and more positive sense of who you are. Being hysterectomized and oophorectomized symbolizes either a gain or a loss. If you view having a hysterectomy as a loss, you might think of yourself as "used goods" or "damaged merchandise." You may come to think of yourself as not being whole, compared with your preconceived ideas. You might dwell on the thought that you are aging or "over the hill." You may focus on your inability to have children. Being hysterectomized and oophorectomized represents for some women a loss of femaleness, a transition to a "unisex" condition, so it is important that you develop a meaning for this surgery, beyond that of your cultural and familial background. Of course, this is a case of deciding whether the glass is half empty or half full. What the experience means is really up to you.

After oophorectomy your major source of estrogen, progesterone, and testosterone is gone. This means that you will need to supplement your body's supply in order to control your moods, cognition, energy level, sexual functioning, and sense of well-being. Also, you will need hormone replacement to prevent such serious physical conditions as heart disease, osteoporosis, and vaginal and urinary problems.

Women who have had their ovaries removed report the following symptoms:

- Fatigue
- Headaches
- Significant hot flushes
- Joint and bone pain
- Dry skin
- Change in vaginal sensation
- Lowered sexual drive and arousal
- Loss of vaginal lubrication with sexual arousal
- Painful intercourse

After oophorectomy, hormone replacement becomes a medical challenge. Finding the proper types and doses of estrogen that fit the particular women may require considerable experimentation. You may not be able to receive hormone replacement for other medical reasons, and the task becomes even more daunting.

Since about 35 percent of women who undergo oophorectomy report not having been adequately prepared for dealing with postmenopausal symptoms, it is important to consider how you get ready for this experience. It may be necessary to begin hormone replacement therapy in advance of the surgery. Psychological preparation is important also, since the removal of your ovaries may have deep and significant meaning to you as a woman.

PMS AND PERIMENOPAUSAL
SYMPTOMS AFTER HYSTERECTOMY
OR PARTIAL OOPHORECTOMY

Another common misunderstanding about hysterectomy relates to menopause. Many people who talk about hysterectomy are really referring to the removal of the ovaries, not just the uterus. If, before the menopause, you are hysterectomized but still have one or both of your ovaries intact, you will continue to have premenstrual and perimenopausal symptoms. You will still have the rhythms of the ovaries, and you will go through the perimenopause and menopause naturally. It is only when you have a complete oophorectomy that you experience surgically induced menopause. If you have a hysterectomy only, you are still likely to approach menopause more rapidly than otherwise, because of the reduced blood supply to the ovaries. Researchers have estimated that there is about a 60 percent chance that you will stop having periods within three to five years. During that time, however, you will continue to have some of the perimenopausal symptoms detailed in Chapter 8.

After hysterectomy, the ovaries have less blood supplied to them. This can cause a decrease in the secretion of estrogen, progesterone, and testosterone. As a consequence, it may be necessary to replace some of these hormones. There may also be an endocrine function in the uterus that is presently unknown. Although you will not be having periods, you will be experiencing premenstrual or perimenopausal symptoms, but perhaps at different levels of intensity. Chapters 7 and 8 describe these symptoms.

Evidence shows that being hysterectomized may lessen premenstrual tension, including such mood states as irritability, anxiety, and depression. Some women, however, report that the procedure did not improve their mood and that their premenstrual symptoms continued. Given these different views of the impact on menstrual cycle functioning, it may be best to observe your own responses in order to validate your own experience. Your consciousness of premenstrual and perimenopausal symptoms may be lessened, since your periods no longer trigger your awareness of your cycles. You can maintain your sense of cyclicity by keeping a symptom calendar, such as those in Chapters 7 and 8.

Hysterectomy, oophorectomy, the onset of menses, abortion, mastectomy, pregnancy, and the cessation of menses are highly significant life events that require adequate coping mechanisms. If you view these occurrences as essentially positive, you are likely to have more resources available to you for dealing with them. Viewing these changes negatively takes energy. Being anxious, angry, or depressed siphons your emotional stamina. You may be adding to your difficulties by the sense you are making of them. Be realistic about the journey that lies ahead. You can reframe any significant life experience so that it nurtures your development rather than having the event impede your ability to change with it. Going through significant physical changes can be complex. They may affect you both emotionally and physiologically, and their emotional effects may be far greater than you anticipate. You may not be able to handle them simply by modifying the ways you view them. Talking with peers may not be enough. You should consider consulting with professionals if you are uncertain about your ability to manage yourself through these transitions. We discuss coping strategies in Chapter 13.

sex and zest:
The possibilities

*"Women are as old as they feel—
and men are old when they lose their feelings."*

— Mae West

BOTH PMS and perimenopause impact your sex life. Changes in sexual desire, arousal, and behavior commonly occur throughout the phases of your menstrual cycle. Following are the stories of four women who are concerned with how their ovarian hormones are affecting them sexually.

> *Phyllis* is twenty-six, a bank clerk. She is in a committed relationship with a young man who is a sales representative. They have enjoyed an active sex life together for the past two years. He has been helping her to become aware of a pattern in which she withdraws from him during the premenstrual phase of her cycles. She often does not know when her period is about to begin, but he can predict it very well. He complains that she will not let him touch her in general, especially sexually. He says that she becomes

moody and "crabby" and that she snaps at him for no apparent reason. She is concerned that for the first time she is having a lower sex drive. This change is beginning to put stress on their relationship. She wonders whether this is "normal," whether something is wrong with her, or whether she is simply "weird."

Harriet is thirty-one, and she is on oral contraceptives. She and her husband are partners in an architectural firm. They have no children yet, but they plan to in the future, as soon as their business grows to the level at which she can afford time off. They are best friends, and they are open about almost everything but sex. She grew up in a home in which neither menses nor sex was ever mentioned. He also grew up in a home in which his parents let him learn about sex only from books. In general, her sex drive is low, and since going on a new pill she has little or no desire for sex. She wants closeness, but every time she asks for it, he interprets the request as a sexual overture. His way of being intimate is intercourse, but her way is through foreplay, romance, and "cuddling." During her premenstrual times the conflict intensifies. She wants more closeness, but she has little desire for genital contact. Just after her periods her drive begins to increase noticeably. It is strongest mid-cycle.

Carlotta is forty-four, in an exclusive relationship with a woman. They have lived together for ten years. She works as department manager in a biotech company, and her partner is a buyer in a retail store. Carlotta is coping with a number of perimenopausal symptoms: low energy, mild depression, generalized aches and pains, vaginal dryness, and mild hair loss. She has enjoyed an active sex life, but recently she complains that her orgasms "take longer." She complains that she does not achieve enough lubrication during sex. She and her partner talk openly about these matters, and they have concluded that as they age they can expect changes such as these. They are committed to look together for treatments that offer promise of symptom relief.

Nicole is forty-nine and married for the past eight years to a stockbroker. She works as a physical therapist at a sports medicine clinic. Her two children from previous marriages live with her. They are sixteen and twenty-three. Her perimenopausal symptoms are relatively new, but she is noticing that her premenstrual symptoms have become more intense. Memory disturbances, abdominal bloating, occasional hot flushes, and restlessness bother her. She feels "on edge" much of the time. She is unable to explain what appears to her to be a burst of sexual interest at some times and almost none at other times. Her husband is confused by this development, and they are considering couples therapy as well as consultation with a physician with expertise in hormonal treatment.

These women present widely different profiles of sexual interest and concerns. Phyllis and Harriet are both having PMS symptoms that affect them sexually. Carlotta and Nicole are going through perimenopause, and it is impacting their sexual functioning. In all four cases, fluctuating hormones are influencing their moods, physical condition, energy level, behavior, and sexual responsiveness. It is common for some oral contraceptives to lower sex drive, but the effect is unique to each woman. With ovarian decline, both during the premenstrual phase of their cycles and during the perimenopausal changes in middle and late adulthood, sexual functioning often declines. This phenomenon is unique to each woman; however, in Nicole's case, there is marked fluctuation in her sexual desire, arousal, and behavior.

In this chapter we present important information about sex from the female point of view, and we offer the premise that while you are undergoing the hormonal changes that PMS and perimenopause bring, sex can become more enjoyable.

WHAT DOES IT MEAN TO BE SEXUAL?

Sex is a complex part of your makeup. Your sexual "apparatus" developed from the time that you were conceived. At that point you were a collection of chromosomes, forming into an embryo that developed ovaries. You began producing female hormones and developing internal and external genitals. As a fetus, your hormonal environment influenced the development of the female brain. Your basic sexual "wiring" was in place at the moment you were born.

Sex encompasses biological, genetic, psychological, and sociocultural aspects. It is expressed as fantasy, desire, arousal, beliefs, attitudes, relationships, and behavior. For most adults sex is a primary force in life. It is tied to your sense of gender (your femaleness) and to intimacy. You may engage in interpersonal sex for a variety of reasons, such as reproduction, recreation, bonding, or tension reduction. You may engage in autosexual stimulation (masturbation) for similar reasons.

Most people think that sexuality begins in adolescence and ends around retirement age. Modern science has established that sexuality actually begins long before birth and continues throughout life. The founder of psychoanalysis, Sigmund Freud, caused a storm of protest when he pointed out that sexuality begins during childhood. In the years following the late nineteenth century, medical and other clinical professionals generally came to accept his postulation as an established fact. Even male fetuses have been observed to experience erections and female ones have shown genital swelling and vaginal lubrication.

During childhood basic attitudes toward sexuality are established. A child learns from adults, the media, and peers what is okay and what is not okay to talk about and do and also learns what is sexually attractive to others. These early experiences become internalized, and they affect the development of your patterns of sexual expression. For example, parents may use special language that makes it clear that your genitals are somehow "bad," and they may even develop euphemisms to describe sexual anatomy and bodily functions. The net result may be that the child learns that erotic pleasure is forbidden because of its connection with "unmentionables." If, on the other hand, parents use proper names for genitalia and communicate openly about sexuality, a child may develop more positive body and self-images and become more receptive to and competent in intimacy and sexual expression.

A young girl learns what it is to be female (and male) and develops an identity based on gender. These models of femaleness and maleness contribute to "baggage" she eventually brings to interpersonal sexuality. She learns what is sexually attractive as she integrates her sense of herself as a female, her understanding of the standards of her society, and her awakening feelings of sexuality. For example, you may be attracted to a person who is similar to you in age, physical characteristics, and cultural background.

During puberty a female experiences many physical, physiological, and social changes. There is an awakening of ovarian and adrenal hormonal development. Puberty can begin as early as age eight or as late as sixteen, and the developmental stage may last from one to six or more years. (See Chapter 5 for more detail on sexual development during this phase.)

So what does love have to do with it? It may be useful to make a distinction between erotic, or passionate, love and companion love. Erotic love is like being "in love." It includes being fixated on the other person, feeling thrilled and even giddy with love, wanting constantly to be with him or her. If, over time, you pair with another person and commit to a long-term, mutually supportive, intimate partnership, you are probably experiencing companion love. This is important for assisting each other in such mutual activities as child rearing, career development, retirement planning, and so on. With either type of love, sex is a way of expressing emotional closeness and of enjoying each other.

Being sexual means being receptive to stimuli in your environment, developing fantasies of pleasure, and taking action to increase your pleasure. Since this cycle of being "triggered," thinking about sex and then taking action, necessarily involves partners, for most women a vital element of being sexual is developing and maintaining quality relationships. There is an analogy between sexual readiness and children's learning readiness. Until a child is ready to learn to read, almost no teaching technique will be effective. When the child becomes "ready" to read, almost any method of teaching will work. Your sexual readiness may work the same way. Until you get yourself into a state of receptivity, or openness, to sexual experience, few stimuli will move you. When you get there, many aspects of your environment may trigger sexual fantasies. A number of things can block or hinder your sexual readiness. For example, you may be reluctant to engage in sex because of an inability or unwillingness to develop a close relationship with a partner, or you may be experiencing guilt about having or fantasizing having sex with someone other than your partner. You may be behaving on the basis of old ideas, such as sex being forbidden or "dirty." You may also be concerned over changes that are occurring in your body as a result of the hormonal fluctuations that accompany the aging process.

SEX IS AN INTEGRAL PART OF SELF

Is it really all genital? Being sexual means expressing yourself in many ways that are not clearly genital. Your total body expression can signal your sexuality to others. Your clothes, your manner of movement, your verbalizations, and your overall demeanor toward others, especially potential sex partners, may communicate this. You may wear clothes that emphasize your figure or that insulate you from being looked at sexually. You may walk suggestively or demurely. Your language may include sexual content, such as jokes or allusions to body functions, or you may be conservative in how you talk. Your nonverbal responses to others may indicate an openness to sexual content and expression, or you may be easily embarrassed or shy about sex. You may be flirtatious and comfortably seductive, or you may be reserved.

Whether you are sexually active or not, you are still a sexual human being, and you will still have sexual responses in the form of fantasies, urges, desires, and reactions. Even celibate adults, who do not engage in either self-stimulation or interpersonal sex, are nonetheless sexual. They simply choose to transcend overt expression. The media bombard us with sexual content, innuendo, and sexual connections almost without end. We see and hear sexual references frequently in advertisements, entertainment shows, and even news broadcasts. Advertisers link sexual pleasure with an incredible array of products, from automobiles to food, household goods, beverages, clothes, and cosmetics. It is probably impossible to live in modern society without becoming influenced by these connections. Your sexual life inevitably reflects the persuasiveness of sexuality in the media. For some people sex appears to have little or no significance. Andy Warhol said, "Sex is the biggest nothing of all time." While he may have been suppressing his sexuality, or he may have experienced difficulty with intimacy, it is equally plausible that he simply concluded that being sexual was unimportant. On the other hand, some entertainers seem preoccupied with expressing themselves as seductive and sexually active. Mae West had a reputation for openness about sex. She defined it this way: "Sex is emotion in motion."

SEXUAL PRACTICES

When you think of sex, what comes to mind? Most people think of sex as intercourse between female and male. In actuality, sexual expression can take many forms, and sexual gratification can be achieved in many ways. Sexuality can be acted out autosexually, heterosexually, homosexually, bisexually, or in a host of "paraphilic" ways. The paraphilias include a wide array of sexual expressions that are considered unconventional, such as fetishes, exhibitionism, and other "unusual" methods of achieving sexual arousal.

Research indicates that the average woman engages in sexual intercourse about six times per month, and the average male has about seven such experiences per month. Surveys of women from late adolescence to the mid-forties strongly indicate a preference for sexual intercourse as a preferred mode: about 80 percent rate the preference as "strong," and most others "somewhat strong." Over 90 percent of women in their mid-forties to late fifties preferred sexual intercourse over alternatives. Just watching a partner undress is very appealing to people from late adolescence to the mid-forties.

The frequency of genital sexual practices within couples varies according to types of relationships. Following are the most common estimates of sexual practices, according to researchers, by type of couple:

- **Heterosexual, married.** Sex about once a week, on the average. After ten years, about half are having sex at least weekly.
- **Heterosexual, co-habitating.** Sex three to four times a week. More sex than heterosexual married couples, regardless of how long they are together.
- **Gay male.** More sex than other types of couples in the early part of their relationship, but less than heterosexual married couples after ten years.
- **Lesbian.** Less sexual activity by far than other types of couples throughout their relationship. See themselves as more sexually compatible than do heterosexual women.

The most common nonintercourse modes of sexual expression include oral-genital sex (cunnilingus and fellatio), masturbation, manual genital stimulation, and anal sex. About two-thirds of women engage in fellatio sometime during their lives, with over 70 percent receiving cunnilingus. About 20 percent of women admit to having anal sex sometime during their lives. Women tend either to strongly like or strongly dislike oral sex. Among women aged eighteen to forty-nine, about 40 percent report that they masturbated in the past year, and about 10 percent say that it was within the past week. Younger women masturbate less than older ones. Women begin at an older age than men do, often after they have had interpersonal sex.

Satisfaction from oral sex varies according to sexual orientation. Following are the most common findings regarding oral sex, according to researchers:

- **Heterosexual male.** Giving or receiving oral sex is related to satisfaction with their sex life and their relationship.
- **Heterosexual female.** Neither giving nor receiving oral sex is necessary for sexual or relationship satisfaction.
- **Gay male.** Important to satisfaction with their sex life. The more they have oral sex, the more satisfied they are.
- **Lesbian.** Those who have oral sex are happier, whether giving or receiving.

The difficulty with establishing reliable statistics is, of course, due to the ability of people to remember and their willingness to report their sexual practices truthfully.

THE SEXUAL CYCLE

Sexual responsiveness takes place in a cyclical sequence. That is, you go through one or more stages in a typical sexual experience. The common steps are:

1. **Desire**   The stimulation of sexual interest.
2. **Excitement**   Genital arousal.
3. **Plateau**   Peaking of arousal.
4. **Orgasm**   Rhythmic muscular contractions.
5. **Resolution**   Return to the unaroused state.

Sexual desire emerges in response to intimacy and trust between you and your partner, and certain smells, food, visual stimuli, memories, images, and so on. This stage is both mental and physical. You have a particular set of sexual motivators, coming from your childhood and previous experiences, and these trigger desire in ways that are unique to you.

The excitement stage means feeling "turned on" or "hot." Your genitals prepare themselves to engage in sexual behavior. Blood flow to your genitals increases, causing the vagina to lubricate, the inner two-thirds of the vagina to expand, the outer lips of the vulva to open, the inner lips to enlarge, and the clitoris to swell. Your nipples may become erect, your heart rate and breathing rates increase, you experience more skin sensitivity, and you have more muscle tension.

During the plateau stage your muscle tension peaks, arousal intensifies, you may get a rash-like reddening on the neck and chest, your heart and breathing rates continue to rise, and your blood pressure increases. The outer one-third of the vagina swells and narrows its opening, the inner two-thirds of the vagina balloons, lifting the cervix and uterus (unless there has been a hysterectomy) away from the end of the vagina. The clitoris and labia continue to enlarge. Your areola, surrounding your nipples, may swell, making it appear that the nipples are not erect, and your breasts may increase in size.

If you enter the orgasm stage, it may last only a few seconds, shorter than the other stages. An orgasm consists of three to ten rhythmic muscular contractions, less than a minute apart. The contractions occur in the outer one-third of the vagina and the uterus and anal areas. You may feel pleasant sensations in your clitoris and overall genital area. An orgasm may come from many kinds of stimulation, but often from stimulation of the clitoris, the vagina, or the "G spot," which is an area of heightened sexual responsiveness on the anterior wall of your vagina. Multiple orgasms within one sexual episode occur less frequently than do single ones. This phenomenon involves re-entering the plateau stage after each orgasm. About one in eleven women report experiencing multiple orgasms.

The resolution stage immediately follows orgasm (or the plateau stage, if you do not experience orgasm). This is the time that the body takes to resume its condition prior to your experiencing the first stage, excitement. During the resolution stage you may feel contented, pleasant, and "cuddly," and you may have a prolonged sense of well-being.

HORMONAL/BIOCHEMICAL CHANGES AND SEXUAL FUNCTIONING

Sexual functioning incorporates desire, arousal, behavior, and satisfaction. Sexual desire and arousal are commonly referred to as sexual "motivators." There are many things that contribute to your sexual desire and arousal. The best evidence seems to indicate wide individual differences among women regarding how and when they become interested in sex and how they express that interest. You may become interested at any point in your menstrual cycle, and you may or may not become aroused sufficiently to motivate you to engage in sexual activity.

In the past researchers have produced conflicting evidence regarding the relationship between the menstrual cycle and sexual activity. There has been a controversy in this area of research for about sixty years. Recent research has found that most women experience increased sexual desire around the expected ovulation date, during the ovulatory phase of the menstrual cycle. Though you may, of course, experience sexual desire during any phase of your cycle. This finding of heightened sexual desire during the ovulatory phase suggests that hormonal factors contribute to the development of sexual desire. When testosterone peaks during the ovulatory stage, it seems to motivate sexual activity. Researchers have found that sexual behavior is most frequent during this stage, indicating that testosterone may be stimulating both sexual desire and arousal.

Estrogen, testosterone, and progesterone play different roles in promoting sexual desire and arousal for women with fully functional ovaries. Estrogen seems to have a largely indirect role. It promotes vaginal and genital health, facilitates vaginal lubrication, promotes nipple sensitivity, and enhances both mood and level of energy—all contributing to sexual desire and arousal. Testosterone is a prime sexual motivator. It promotes sexual drive and fantasies and has a direct effect on sexual arousal. These two hormones, estrogen and testosterone, in combination produce much of what you experience as sexual desire and arousal. Progesterone, in a sense, works against the effects of estrogen and testosterone with regard to sexual desire and arousal. It dampens sexual desire, decreases energy, lowers your mood, increases your irritability, and generally makes engaging in sexual activity less likely (see Chapter 2).

If you are experiencing PMS, the severity of your symptoms may make sex less attractive during the luteal phase of your cycle. On the other hand, some women report that their sexual desire peaks one or two days before menstruation and continues during the menstrual phase. Clearly more research is needed here, since the situation seems to be unique for each woman. If your PMS symptoms include irritability, increase in arguments with your partner(s), depression, social withdrawal, or anxiety, you are less likely to find a willing partner for sexual activity. Sexual activity, on the other hand, may provide relief for you during this phase of your cycle. If your PMS symptoms cause you to burden other people with your problems, you may carry a sense of guilt or remorse when the symptoms subside. This could result in your becoming reluctant to engage in intimate encounters, including sexual ones. The condition may not, however, prevent engaging in masturbation.

For perimenopausal women the reduction in hormones secreted by aging ovaries can affect sexual functioning. During this developmental period you establish most of the sexual norms that are likely to determine your sexual experience after the menopause. Regular sexual activity helps maintain vaginal health, increases the blood supply to vaginal tissues, increases lubrication, and retards genital atrophy. It becomes a matter of "use it or lose it." However, as aging occurs, sexual activity alone without hormonal intervention will not ensure that you will maintain sexual desire and arousal. Since both estrogen and testosterone gradually decline during perimenopause, your sexual motivation is likely to become erratic. Some women report that they need different sexual stimulation, that they take longer to climax, and that their orgasms are different in intensity than before. For some women sexual desire increases during this time of their lives. This may be related to lifestyle changes (e.g., new partner, more time available, and so on) or ovarian changes. The fluctuation of ovarian hormones causes the body to compensate, and this can result in an increase in both estrogen and testosterone (see Chapter 2). In addition, some women who are undergoing hormone replacement therapy report that "sex is better than ever."

DYSFUNCTIONS

For some women sex is something to be avoided. This feeling can come from several causes, such as a history of sexual abuse, rape, or other sexual assault; being vulnerable to depression or anxiety; being in an unsatisfying relationship; having medical conditions that interfere; using medications that influence sexuality; lack of education about sex; inability to communicate effectively about sex; or having a lack of time. Some women believe that sex stops at a certain age. Others feel trapped or bored in their relationship with their sex partner. Women who engage in extramarital sex may worry about sexually transmitted diseases, including AIDS.

There are several sets of sexual disorders that require clinical treatment. The major categories are:

- **Desire disorders.** These include difficulties with producing sexual fantasies and having little or no sexual desire, and extreme aversion to or avoidance of any genital sexual contact with a partner.

- **Arousal disorder.** Persistent inability to lubricate sufficiently or have genital swelling and the lack of excitement or pleasure in sexual activity.

- **Orgasmic disorder.** Persistent delay or absence of orgasm following normal arousal.

- **Painful disorders.** Recurrent or persistent genital pain before, during, or after sexual intercourse. Recurrent or persistent involuntary spasm of the external vaginal muscles.

- **Other disorders.** Inability to feel erotic sensations, even when able to have orgasms; the female equivalent to the male disorder, premature ejaculation; genital pain during masturbation; feelings of inadequacy regarding genitals, performance, self-imposed standards of femininity; distress over seeing others as sexual conquests; persistent and marked distress about one's sexual orientation.

Treatment for these sexual dysfunctions can involve both medical and psychotherapeutic interventions. The first step, of course, is a complete medical and psychological assessment. It is estimated that over half of the female population experiences one or more sexual dysfunctions sometime during their lives. In the next chapter we will discuss a number of options available to women who may be suffering from these difficulties.

SEX CAN GET BETTER

We have been discussing sex primarily in terms of desire and arousal, along with references to sexual behavior. Of course, the desired result is satisfaction, not just activity. Standards for sexual satisfaction are unique to each woman. You may be satisfied with experiencing emotional closeness, regardless of whether you achieve orgasm. You may require yourself to have an orgasm. You may be satisfied with feeling "turned on," whether it is with a partner or not. You may only be satisfied if somehow you please your partner. You may require variety in your sexual practices as a necessary ingredient for satisfaction. Any of these criteria could be a trap. Placing undue demands on yourself may make you unnecessarily vulnerable to dissatisfaction when "things don't go right," particularly with a partner. Having better sex may begin with challenging your personal expectations and standards. If you are able to become flexible in expressing yourself sexually, you might have more fun and be more desirable.

Fantasy and foreplay are central to a satisfying sexual experience. Your imagination can greatly enhance your excitement and arousal. Becoming comfortable with producing sexual imagery can make sexual activities richer and more fulfilling. Sometimes fantasy is deemed as daydreaming or idle thinking. Fantasy can be used as a stimulus for both self-sex and activities with a partner.

You may or may not share your fantasy material with your sex partner. You might imagine pleasurable sexual activities, partners, past sex partners, or situations that you have never experienced. You might even fantasize "forbidden acts."

Foreplay consists of the things that you and a partner do to heighten arousal. Some of these activities may include such things as kissing, stroking and massaging, talking, reading erotic material, or using visual materials. Older women need more foreplay, since both arousal and orgasmic functioning take longer. People differ with regard to their general interest in sexuality, and some have less need for being sexual than others have. People with lower sexual appetites probably require additional time in foreplay activities. People with high sexual appetites may need to slow down a bit in order to be sensitive to their sex partners.

There are numerous things that you can experiment with to increase sexual pleasure. If you have a partner, you might discuss likes and dislikes and play with different ways of pleasing each other. You may also exchange and co-create sexual fantasies. You can use various "sex toys" to increase the variety in your lovemaking activities. You may find that sexually explicit material, such as romantic novels, magazines, videos, and movies, may increase erotic pleasure for you.

Evidence shows that both younger and single people take more time during interpersonal sex. You may need to talk with your partner(s) about your needs with regard to the timing of a sexual encounter. It is okay to request that your partner take your particular rhythm into account during the experience.

Sex is a important indicator of satisfaction in relationships. There is a correlation between frequency of sexual satisfaction and conflict in heterosexual married and gay male couples. Those with more conflict tend not to have satisfying sex lives. Lesbians, on the other hand, do not feel unsatisfied with infrequent sex. Lesbians report that they find satisfaction in nongenital ways, such as cuddling, touching, stroking, and kissing.

In Chapter 9 we emphasize the need for openness between partners about sex. Chapter 13 provides suggestions for working on relationships. In addition, we will include information on hormone replacement therapy. Both practices can enhance your ability to enjoy yourself sexually.

12

The Beauty of Aging

"I'm tired of all this nonsense about beauty being only skin-deep. That's deep enough. What do you want, an adorable pancreas?"

—Jean Kerr

All women approach aging differently. Some fear its changes, and others "go with the flow." Consider these two:

> *Mae* is in her mid-forties, and she is active in both her church and community activities as a volunteer. Her four children range in age from eight to sixteen. She is a homemaker, and her twenty-year marriage is still fun. Taking care of her physical fitness is a priority for Mae. She walks and jogs with friends, and about once a week she lifts weights at the gym. She pays a lot of attention to her weight and physical appearance. She goes to a skin-care salon every week or so for a facial or massage, and she get her nails done regularly. She is constantly on the lookout for new cosmetics and skin products that may enhance her youthfulness. She is getting new wrinkles, but

she is secretly saving for plastic surgery. She frequently shops for the latest fashions when they are on sale. Her husband, who likes her to accompany him to social functions, is enthralled with her physical appearance, but he complains about how much her upkeep is costing him. She feels pressure to remain "young-looking" for him, even though he has never said that he wants her to remain young.

Nancy is also in her mid-forties, and she is enjoying life these days. She is single, and she frequently dates several men. She sees herself as a "free spirit," and she now looks back at her former marriages as times when she had compromised to meet others' expectations. Her new wrinkles are a sign that she is maturing, and she is less bothered than glad at becoming a bit wiser as she ages. She has recently taken a course in sculpture, and one of her male friends is teaching her golf. Her work as a firefighter is both dangerous and exciting, and she has hopes of promotion soon. She keeps the gray out of her hair but attempts to look as natural as possible. Since she is unable to conceive, she is not concerned about the ticking of her "biological clock." She has thought about adopting a child, but she decided not to do this as a single parent, and she is reluctant to give up personal freedom in the process. She is under the care of a homeopath who is working to keep her skin alive and her emotions in balance.

These two women approach their aging very differently. Mae is resisting becoming older, and she is desperately attempting to maintain youthfulness. Mae's pleasure may lie in remaining attractive at all costs. She may, however, be caught up in a lifestyle that requires her to fight aging. She does not seem to know how to look within herself and make choices that might free her to develop her own expectations instead of trying always to please others. On the other hand, Nancy views her situation as a natural series of developments that are not interfering with her basic enjoyment of herself and others. She is focused on herself and has built a life of self-expression. In her profession clothes are not a part of expressing who she is. Her work activities and her competency in carrying them out are much more important to her. These two women probably have very different answers to the question, "What is beauty?"

As you go through midlife, you may experience many changes. Here are some that women report.

> *I am learning to slow down and enjoy my own pace.*
>
> *I am appreciating the people around me more these days.*
>
> *I can see the effects of gravity on my body. No matter how much I exercise or watch what I eat, aging is upon me.*
>
> *The lines on my face are indicative of my life story, and I am learning to appreciate them.*
>
> *I am listening more to my 'inner voices,' rather than taking care of everyone else.*
>
> *As I mature, I seem to be gaining a sense of inner peace.*
>
> *I am moving away from frantically meeting others' expectations and developing my own priorities.*
>
> *My intimate relationships are complicated and changing.*
>
> *I am wondering whether all of what I am involved in makes sense.*

With aging can come growth in wisdom, balance, perspective, and grace. During midlife, you may experience a resurgence of energy and revitalization that can increase your self-esteem and confidence. Thinking of the processes of aging and how you feel about yourself, however, may be best thought of in terms of mastering the challenges that come with life changes. You embrace the changes that are predictable during midlife and concentrate on keeping yourself attractive *as a person.*

There are no benchmarks for what is happening to women today. You are living longer, and advances in medical science, psychology, and nutrition have stretched your developmental phases out. You are creating the journey as you go along. This requires that you adjust your thinking to new realities. What you need is a model of yourself that incorporates a long life, changing roles, and positive expectations. Your beliefs about yourself and about aging create the realities that you are likely to encounter. If your model of aging calls for you to become less attractive or even infirm, the way you think can actually bring about the conditions that lead to such outcomes. Rather than only searching for youthfulness in a bottle or tube, it may be more important to nurture it within yourself. If you maintain positive mental attitudes toward yourself as your physiology changes, you will project your inner beauty. In other words, what we concentrate on becomes what we live through. We create the reality, and there are apparently few limits on what we can produce through our thinking.

Some women dread aging. As they approach a birthday that ends in zero (thirty, forty, fifty), they either deny that they are, in fact, aging, or they simply do not want to talk about it with anyone. This silent fear can take its toll, both physically and psychologically. What women dread or fear usually includes irreversible physical and mental deterioration, loss of productivity, change in relationships, loss of physical attractiveness, and loneliness. For the average person, midlife is the time in which you face for the first time your mortality. This existential condition requires you to face the fact that you will always ultimately be alone. As you continue to live through the rest of your years, you will be responsible for whatever happens to you. It will be up to you to remain happy and productive.

Cynics sometimes remark that "nobody gets out of here alive." The challenges and opportunity of aging are the ability to see them as natural and to accept them as part of living. Wrinkles, sags, and weight gain are simply part of how your body expresses itself as a result of several important changes: your changing physiology, the stresses of everyday living, modifying relationships with others, and managing a career. A song asks, "Is that all there is?" What there is, is an opportunity for you to take personal responsibility for keeping yourself attractive by affirming yourself and by remaining positive as you encounter physical and physiological change.

What Is Beauty?

The dictionary defines beauty as "a combination of all the qualities of a person that delight the senses and please the mind." Cultural standards usually evaluate beauty externally. The media and fashion industry propagandize people into valuing youthful physical perfection. If you think of aging as an inevitable decline of youthful appearance, you can get caught in the trap of endlessly searching for the right diet, clothes, cosmetics, and therapies to stop the process. It is easy to get caught in this trap. The cosmetic industry is a multibillion-dollar enterprise, beauty contests abound, and cosmetic surgery is increasing steadily.

Advertisers lead us to believe that beauty comes out of a bottle or tube and that it can be purchased. Generally, both women and men use more products as they age, with women's use significantly higher. Clinique/Marie Claire's 1996 survey found that 92 percent of women felt that cosmetic or beauty products are important in maintaining physical attractiveness. The same survey found that 72 percent were concerned with looking older, but only 10 percent felt anxious about it. The overwhelming majority (92 percent) said that they wanted to look the best they can for their age. Studies of attractiveness have shown that even babies respond more positively to people who might be conventionally described as physically attractive. Mothers are more attentive to babies who are physically attractive. Each of us is judged instantaneously according to our physical presentations. Standards of beauty become internalized. These standards slowly change as we age. To assist yourself in adopting new images of aging, you might search for new models of women who are your age or older and who have the kind of inner beauty that attracts you. There is evidence that American women are becoming less concerned about the effects of aging and less willing to do whatever it takes to retain a youthful look. The new emphasis is on doing the best you can with what you have. This notion challenges the dominant sociocultural value that emphasizes physical attractiveness as being youth-related.

Beauty becomes more than physical appearance. Inner beauty, independent of physical presentation, is ageless. It involves confidence, vitality, energy, learning, growth, playfulness, and a carefree disposition. It is important to shift your view of beauty away from the "fresh look of youth." Beauty centers on how you think about yourself and how you behave. Your lifestyle and self-expression become the basis for your attractiveness. This does not mean that you "let yourself go," neglecting your physical appearance altogether. It simply means that you concentrate on being a beautiful person in a body that is changing. The feeling is transcendent. You go beyond preoccupation with your appearance and choose your own inner strength and expressiveness. If you are "going with the flow," you may be able to see that as powerful and beautiful in its own way. Taking personal responsibility to leading a fulfilling life is a way of showing your beauty to the world.

PAYOFFS OF PHYSICAL BEAUTY

"Being beautiful" does not necessarily mean that you have to live up to your and others' expectations constantly. If you are trapped by the need for others' approval, you will not learn how to appreciate those aspects of yourself that are, in fact, beautiful. Many people "discount" their positive qualities. They are even embarrassed by positive feedback from others. It is important to develop the capability of affirming your positive qualities, whether they are noticed by others or not.

"Being beautiful" gets you attention. If you are one of the "beautiful people," others may be drawn to you, admire you, and expect more from you. If the basis of your beauty is primarily your physical presentation, you will likely gain much attention in the forms of social and sexual advances. These reactions can cause you to feel empowered and alive or exposed and vulnerable. You might believe that you have to keep up the act or else people might go away. Physical beauty can evoke envy or resentment among other women.

People who do not fit cultural stereotypes of the beautiful woman as displayed on billboards, in TV commercials, and beauty magazines may feel inferior and develop a more negative sense of self. Women who hold this view of beauty can come to feel intensely resentful toward other women. This can generate feelings of aloneness and vulnerability, which can come about from a lack of female companionship. As women age, they can lose some of this sense of competitiveness and share with others in more fulfilling ways.

If your notion of beauty is being able to interact well with others socially, the aging process will empower you. It may be easier for you to sustain this way of expressing yourself rather than attempt to remain youthful looking. This way involves strengthening your self-regard and letting yourself become more assertive, powerful, energetic, and flowing.

SELF-REGARD, BODY IMAGE, AND SELF-IMAGE

You have a "working image," or concept, of what your body looks like. We call this your body image. You have a sense of the kind of person you are, and we call that your self-image. Finally, you have a state of being in which you have feelings about yourself, and we term that your self-esteem or self-regard. You might think of your self-regard as your "inner mirror," what is reflected back to your consciousness as you meditate on who you are. Your concept of yourself is fluid, and it can turn positive or negative as you make sense out of what happens within and around you. You can change your self-concept by affirming your strengths and acknowledging opportunities to improve yourself. You can strengthen your self-regard by claiming your successes (even small, unobserved ones) and your personal strengths. Since a key component of your self-regard is your physical appearance, it is important to find ways of re-evaluating yourself as aging induces changes in your anatomy, physiology, and psychology.

How you conceptualize the ideal body is a significant aspect of your sense of beauty. Since you have been subjected to a barrage of conditioning that portrays the ideal female body as youthful and thin, you may need to consciously let go of this notion in order to realize your own potential. If you remain stuck in the culturally defined model, the aging process will be frustrating.

You might attempt to redefine beauty in other terms. Some women use such criteria as muscularity, roundedness, softness, fluidity, and so on.

Being attractive means thinking you are attractive and acting in ways that are pleasing to yourself and others. Your body is only one part of you. Other parts are thinking, behavior, feelings, values, skills, and knowledge. Your body gives you many important cues that can assist you in finding your way in the world. If you become "disconnected" from your body sensations, this may result in difficulties with decision making and in making sense of your changing emotions and cognitions. It is important, then, that you monitor your sensations as you decide how to act.

How you define *yourself* is foundational. You have an image of yourself that formed in early childhood, and it came from the reactions of others to you. When a stranger asks you who you are, you will likely respond in terms of the work you do or some other aspect of your living situation, such as who your spouse is, whether you have children, where you live, and so on. What is more important is how you define yourself in terms of your values, competencies, needs, wants, desires, and preferences. Developing a holistic sense of who you are, what you stand for, where you are going, and the difference you want to make in the world are highly valuable quests. You need to integrate these views of yourself into how you see your body also. In other words, if someone asks you, you might say (at least to yourself), "I am a woman who values openness, who takes reasonable risks, who gains satisfaction in her children's development, and who is working on remaining healthy and fit." Such an image would balance the duality of mind and body into a personally meaningful statement.

Our self-images come from many sources. We develop our understandings of ourselves from growing up in a cultural mix, by taking on some of the tenets of the dominant religion during childhood, and assuming our places in the histories of our families. As our personalities unfold, we create a working image of who we are. When we begin to undergo physiological changes, such as during puberty, PMS, and perimenopause, we modify our self-images to take these new developments into account. If we begin to suffer from some significant medical condition, we also alter our views of ourselves. Various life events can change our sense of who we are, bringing about psychological conditions that may enlighten or debilitate us. We might learn a sense of helplessness, but if we are nurtured well, we create a strong sense of self and cope with the demands of daily growth and development as we encounter them. So, your self-image is a montage of what you have seen, how people have reacted to you, how you have behaved in response to the changes you have experienced, and how you have pieced all this together into a coherent whole.

Your thirties and forties will bring about challenges. Constants that you can rely on are a strong sense of self, a mature view of your body, and careful monitoring of your sensations and reactions to the many symptoms you experience. Your self-esteem and self-image can support you through these changes and not allow you to be overtaken by them.

How to Embrace the Beauty of Aging

There are many things you can do to maintain a positive outlook on PMS and perimenopause. You might experiment with any or all of the following.

Creating a vision of beauty. Take time out to write down your present standards for beauty. If you prefer, sit in a quiet place, close your eyes, and develop a visual image of beauty as you see it. Reflect on the points of this chapter as you go through this exercise.

Claiming inner strengths. Make a list of the things you are good at. You may need to ask others to help you with this project, since you may be "discounting" your competencies ("Everyone can do that"). Alternatively, you might keep a diary of your accomplishments, recording how you personally brought about the desired results.

Learning to listen to body sensations. When you experience a negative emotion, stop and pay careful attention to how your body is reacting. Look for such cues as tension in various parts of your body, flushness, stomach churning, change in breath, and so on. Different emotions may be accompanied by different cues. Your PMS and perimenopause symptoms can be your teachers, and aging can show you different patterns for making choices. Notice subtle changes in your symptoms, so that you can discover how your symptomatology is developing.

Appreciating the power of the mind. You can learn how to reframe situations that you encounter. Pay careful attention to your "shoulds, oughts, musts, and onlys." Your reactions are mediated by the sense that you make out of situations. Making different sense, with difference assumptions and realistic expectations, can release you from some toxic emotions. As you age, you can become more beautiful as you convert experience into wisdom.

Self-affirmations. Repeating phrases that are positive can help you "grow into" them. You may already use favorite sayings to strengthen yourself in difficult times, and you can exchange these with others to enlarge your repertoire. One of the earliest psychotherapists had his patients look in the mirror and repeat, "Every day in every way, I am getting better and better."

Attending to desired outcomes more than immediate pleasure. Part of becoming mature is learning how to engage in "delayed gratification." When you are facing a difficult situation, focus on your goals rather than on simply smoothing out the conflict.

Staying with the feeling. When you become frustrated, angry, tense, or upset, try to concentrate on how the feeling can help you make a decision. Avoid denying, running away from, or otherwise attempting to escape from the feeling. Instead of overeating, compulsively shopping, or abusing substances, for example, acknowledge the feeling and affirm your ability to choose how you will respond. The body changes that are a result of aging give you many opportunities to change how you respond when you are emotional. You become more beautiful as a person as you grow in competence in this area.

Rewarding progress rather than perfection. You may be the only one who knows how difficult a task is to perform, so it is important that you reward yourself for making satisfactory steps toward your goal. Waiting until you have completed the job perfectly makes you unduly vulnerable. You may not even be able to reach the target. Give yourself credit for the many small steps you take that lead you to a desired outcome.

Setting realistic goals. A Robert Browning poem says that "your reach should exceed your grasp." You need to set "stretch" goals, ones that require you to learn and grow, but you need to be careful not to set yourself up for failure by setting your sights so high that you cannot accomplish your aims. Make sure that you establish targets for yourself that are both desirable and doable.

Acknowledging limitations. None of us is perfect. An old saying goes, "Here I am, warts and all." It is important for you to be honest with yourself regarding your personal limitations, without becoming morbid in the process. As you age, you can practice noticing your body changes and welcoming them rather than dreading or devaluing them. Your career may "top out," for example, and you may need to develop other interests that are pleasurable for you.

Focusing on possibilities. This means catching yourself when you sound pessimistic and reversing your thought patterns. The

Chinese characters for change are "danger" and "opportunity." Focus on the latter. When you are faced with conflict, look for positive outcomes that can be achieved by facing it productively.

Beauty is not only skin deep. It is who you totally are, reflecting both your physical presentation and your inner self. Paying attention to both in a balanced way means that you actually grow in beauty as you age.

13

what you can do about pms and perimenopause

*"When you're at the edge of a cliff,
sometimes progress is a step backwards."*

—Anonymous

"If It Is to Be, It's Up to Me"

Your health is your business so it is important to take personal responsibility for working with your PMS and perimenopause, using others as resources. You have to manage your own health care. Health-care professionals are part of *your* team and might include a psychotherapist, nurse practitioner, physician's assistant, acupuncturist, nutritional consultant, naturopath, gynecologist, internal-medicine specialist, reproductive endocrinologist, urologist, masseuse, and chiropractor. Since these providers do not routinely talk with each other about your care, it is up to you to coordinate their communication. You may consult with them for information on your options, but you make decisions based on their advice and your own priorities. Your state of being is no one else's responsibility. The quality of your life is an essential consideration in making decisions about any type of treatment. You need to consider what parts of your life feel out of balance and find out what you can do to change those conditions.

Maintaining your well-being means going through the following steps:

1. **Assess your symptoms.** Work on becoming sensitive to the subtle changes that your body undergoes during your cycle and during your aging process. Pay attention to the onset, intensity, and duration of your symptoms. The worksheets in Chapters 7 and 8 can be used or adapted for recording your symptoms.

2. **Involve others.** Your family, friends, coworkers, physician, psychotherapist, and other health-care providers can give you important information about how they perceive you during your cycle, changes they observe, and treatments that you might consider. Ask for research evidence from those who can provide it.

3. **Consider your options.** If you have any doubts about recommended approaches, seek additional opinions, read, and attend seminars or lectures.

4. **Consider your family history.** Think about your family in terms of both medical and psychological health. Weigh the treatments that you may be considering in the light of this generational health history. Reflect on how you have responded to previous approaches.

5. **Weigh the evidence before deciding.** Remember that there is no "right way" to work with your symptoms. Make your own decisions based on the best informa-

tion that you can gather. Empowering yourself does not mean following others' advice blindly but taking it into account as you commit yourself to action.

6. **Set goals.** Having short- and long-term targets may help you take charge of dealing with PMS and peri-menopause. In general, it is best to make "stretch" goals, ones that require you to reach farther than you ordinarily do. Some of your goals may span the next hour or day, while others may span weeks, months, or even years. Some criteria to bear in mind are those captured in Jones' SPIRO Model:

S Specificity.   What *exactly* are you going to do?
P Performance.   What exactly are you going to *do?*
I Involvement.   What exactly are *you* going to do?
R Realism.   Can it be done, given your resources?
O Observability. How will you know that you have succeeded?

Setting goals may involve creating a vision for yourself. This means writing a statement that describes a way of being that is substantially better than your present condition. The two major considerations for stating your vision should be that it is both desirable and doable.

7. **Forgive yourself.** You may not follow your chosen approach with 100 percent reliability. Your self-improvement program may not give you relief from all your premenstrual or perimenopausal symptoms, and you may experience continuing symptoms even as you attempt to prevent them. All these eventualities can cost you in terms of self-esteem, and your program's success can be jeopardized in the process. It is

important that you forgive yourself when you make mistakes, when you are inconsistent, or when you reach for goals that are unattainable at the time.

8. **Reward yourself.** No one else may know how difficult your self-improvement program is better than you do. They may not notice your progress or the energy you expend in taking care of yourself.

9. **Search for wisdom.** See your mistakes as your great teachers. View your attempts at working through your symptoms as a growth process. Listen to yourself and intuit what is good for you. Search for wisdom from acquaintances and from what you read.

PMS TREATMENTS

Use the symptom rating scale in Chapter 7 to assess your premenstrual symptoms to help you discover patterns and trends. This knowledge can alert you to probable difficulties, and you may be able to manage your well-being better as a result. You may learn how to adjust your approach to the severity levels of your symptoms. Make a calendar of your most common symptoms, as illustrated in Chapter 7, so that you can track your progress in alleviating them.

There is no therapy that has been consistently shown to reduce premenstrual symptoms. Your approach needs to be uniquely designed. Some combination of medical, psychotherapeutic, nutritional, and exercise regimes offers promise of giving you the symptom relief that you might desire. In addition, alternative forms of medical health-care delivery are available for your consideration in devising your particular approach.

Medical Treatments

Physicians have reported success in alleviating premenstrual symptoms with a number of medications. There is no one medication that will treat the entire set of premenstrual symptoms. Specific premenstrual symptoms have been successfully treated with seratonin reuptake inhibitors, such as fluoexetine (Prozac) for anxiety and depression. Some physicians prescribe medications for specific mood disorders, such as anti-anxiety agents or antidepressants. Specific physical symptoms, such as water retention, headaches, and joint aches and pains, may be treated with medications.

Hormonal treatments attempt to adjust the hormonal levels during the menstrual cycle. Your treatment may involve estrogen or progesterone or in combination. The most effective forms are transdermal or skin patches (estradiol), oral estrogen preparations (estradiol or estrone), and pellets that are inserted under the skin by medical personnel. Different forms of estrogen, delivered through these three methods, will produce different effects, so it is necessary to tailor the dose, frequency, and type to the particular needs of a patient. The combination of estrogen and progesterone has been found to be superior to progesterone alone in alleviating premenstrual symptoms. If your progesterone levels are sufficient, estrogen replacement may be all that is needed. If, however, you take estrogen alone and do not produce adequate levels of progesterone naturally, you may run the risk of endometrial cancer. In that case, a carefully controlled regimen of a combination of estrogen and progesterone might be called for. Research suggests that taking progesterone alone is no better than taking a placebo. An alternate form of hormone replacement is oral contraceptives which provide stability of ovarian hormones, predictability in your menstrual cycle, and contraception. These vary in terms of the relative amounts of estrogen and progesterone, so learn which fits your physiology better.

Choosing a medical practitioner is an important step for you. Some criteria to consider are specialty, philosophy, location, gender, age, reputation, and cost. Seek out providers who see health as both mental and physical, who will coordinate with other members of your team, and who will treat you holistically, that is, not just as a physical being.

Psychotherapeutic Treatments

Psychotherapy is beneficial in helping work through your PMS experiences. The focus should be on working with problematic moods and difficulties with cognition, as well as self-regard. Since internal conflicts and external stressors can intensify premenstrual symptoms, working therapeutically with these factors can reduce your symptoms. Psychotherapy may be brief, short-term, or long-term, depending on the complexity of your total situation.

Psychotherapy is used to treat depression, anxiety, anger, and other problems with moods. The most effective forms of psychotherapy for PMS combine cognitive-behavioral (e.g., cognitive restructuring) with psychodynamic therapy. This involves helping you decipher your thinking patterns, "tease out" whatever irrational thoughts you may have developed, explore the origins of your psychological condition, and equip you with methods and thought processes that can enable you to cope with PMS effectively. Treatment with medications such as antidepressants and anti-anxiety agents is also used to reduce premenstrual symptoms. Both types of treatment—psychotherapy and medications—are sometimes required. Assertiveness and relaxation training have also benefited many women in obtaining relief from mood and interpersonal difficulties.

Group psychotherapy can provide an opportunity to learn from others, gain support for your self-management of PMS, and help you maintain your commitment to improving your personal well-being. Typically, groups consist of women who are concerned about their PMS experiences and its impact on their daily lives and relationships. Research has indicated that this form of therapy is effective in helping women reduce their premenstrual symptoms.

Choosing a psychotherapist is an important step. Since you will need to be completely open with this person, think about the qualities and qualifications of that health-care provider before committing to the relationship. Some criteria to consider are specialty, general approach, location, gender, age, reputation, and cost.

Nutritional Treatments

Nutrition should be an important part of each woman's treatment program. Research indicates that what you eat and drink can affect your premenstrual symptoms significantly, either positively or negatively. Overeating, consuming excessive alcohol, and taking stimulants such as caffeine can cause your system to compensate and may increase the severity of your premenstrual symptoms in the process. You have less resistance to stress, and you may have an increased desire for sweets and fast foods. Poor nutrition can also result in a loss of self-esteem and less commitment to taking care of yourself generally. Consuming sweets and junk food may increase your seratonin level rapidly and increase your blood sugar, resulting in a quick onset of drowsiness, nervousness, and other negative symptoms. Paying attention to your nutrition may be one of the very best ways of treating yourself. It is not so much a matter of finding the best diet for you, but one of changing your nutritional lifestyle altogether.

Nutritional treatments often emphasize a particular mix of proteins (lean meats, fowl, fish, soy products), complex carbohydrates (fruits, vegetables, grains, pasta), and fats (oils, butter, or margarine) to control premenstrual symptoms. Eating a lot of complex carbohydrates, together with proteins, can reduce water retention, improve mood, and raise your energy level. Eating about every three to four hours in small amounts can regulate your blood sugar more readily than eating the traditional "three squares" each day. This blood sugar control helps regulate your mood and some of the physical premenstrual symptoms, such as cravings.

While managing your PMS, your diet should contain little or no caffeine (including that in chocolate). Your consumption of alcohol should be in small amounts, if at all. Both wine and beer have the ability to enhance the production of estradiol, but they can negatively affect your blood sugar level if you consume great amounts. Avoid consuming simple sugars, such as sweets, since they can decrease your blood sugar control. Emphasize complex carbohydrates in your diet, including vegetables, legumes, whole grains, pasta, and brown rice. Avoid fatty foods, since your fat total should not exceed 15 to 30 percent of your total caloric intake. Reduce your animal-fat intake, but make sure that you get enough protein (fish, poultry, and soy products). It is still true that you should drink about eight glasses of water each day. Small, frequent meals and snacks help to control blood sugar. Avoid going more than twelve hours without food at night. Control your sodium intake to contribute to cardiovascular fitness. Your diet should be high in fiber (e.g., cereals, grains, etc.) and contain the essential fatty acids (e.g., safflower oil, sunflower oil, black currant seed oil, etc.).

In summary, you can prevent some PMS discomfort and strengthen your overall physical health by following the guidelines in Table 13-1:

FOODS TO CONSUME	FOODS TO AVOID
Fruits	Products high in refined sugar
Fresh vegetables	Alcohol (in excess)
Whole grains	Caffeinated substances, such as
Lean meats	coffee, black tea, and chocolate
Fowl	Fatty meats
Fish	Deep-fried foods
Soy products	Processed fats
Brown rice	Fast foods
Pasta	Foods high in sodium
Potatoes	
Yams	
Seeds	
Nuts	
Vegetable or seed oil	
Low- or nonfat dairy products	
Water	
Decaffeinated tea and coffee	

Table 13-1

Vitamin and mineral supplements can help to correct deficiencies in your food intake. Although there is considerable debate about this practice, there is general agreement that you should take a multivitamin and multimineral supplement daily for PMS. In addition, you should take magnesium, vitamins C, E, and B complex, a source of essential fatty acids.

Herbal treatments are available for PMS as well. There are conflicting claims about the efficacy of these preparations, but they are widely used throughout the world. Here are some herbal potions that women use to treat their PMS symptoms, along with claims about their effects:

Dong quai. This herb equalizes high and low levels of estrogen. It has beneficial cardiovascular effects by dilating blood vessels and decreases clotting. Women with heavy flow, fibroids, or diarrhea should avoid this herb.

Vitex. This herb normalizes the menstrual cycle and increases the levels of estrogen and progesterone. It is used to regulate menstrual bleeding and shrink fibroids.

Black cohosh root. This potion, an estrogenic substance, helps to stimulate the ovarian secretion of estrogen, progesterone, and testosterone. Other effects include a decrease in water retention, improvement of digestion, and calmness. The use of this potion can cause heavy flow.

Other herbs are used to treat specific PMS symptoms. For anxiety and depression some women use skullcap, wild oats, wood betony, vervain, and chamomile. For extreme tension and irritability valerian passionflower is sometimes used. For water retention, breast tenderness, and bloating some women use dandelion leaf, corn silk, and burdock. For breast tenderness some use cleavers, pokeroot, and calendula.

Exercise Treatments

This form of treatment, or lifestyle practice, has been found to improve premenstrual symptoms. Exercise can elevate your mood by naturally enhancing the release of endorphins, increase your self-regard, enhance muscle strength, increase bone mass, and improve your overall health. Since exercise affects your brain chemistry (see Chapter 2), it appears to be linked to the ovarian and adrenal hormones. Being physically active, which includes engaging in aerobic exercise for at least thirty minutes three to four times per week, can modify the severity of your premenstrual symptoms. You may choose to consult with a personal trainer to develop an exercise regimen that is tailored to your fitness. A trainer can teach you proper exercise methods and how to avoid injury.

Alternative Treatments

There is little scientific research evidence regarding these therapies in relation to treating PMS symptoms. These forms of health care may alleviate specific symptoms, however. Here is a brief definition of the more common alternative treatment disciplines:

Acupuncture. This is a form of Chinese medicine that employs needles that are inserted into the body along its meridians and manipulated to unblock and balance the body's energy flow. The method is intended to relieve pain through regional anesthesia. Acupuncturists often combine Chinese herbs and homeopathy (see below) with their treatment.

Chiropractic. This discipline focuses on manipulation of the vertebrae of the spine and other body structures. Adjustments can lead to improved balance, less pain, and lowered tension. The cause of disease is treated as an abnormal functioning of the nervous system.

Homeopathy. This discipline searches for "mimicking" curative substances, ones that match the negative body conditions, in a manner similar to inoculation in traditional medicine. The homeopath administers minute dosages of substances that in large amounts could produce symptoms of the disease under treatment. The goal is not to suppress symptoms but to enable the body to heal itself.

Massage and body work. This approach takes myriad forms, all of which emphasize improving circulation and relaxation of the mind and body. Most approaches feature rubbing or kneading the body in order to relax the muscles and relieve tension. The premise is that removing stress from the body prevents chronic illness and disease.

Reflexology. This form of massage focuses on pressure points in the feet and hands that correspond to parts of the body that may be causing negative symptoms. The method relieves nervous tension through finger pressure.

Naturopathy. This discipline combines treatment methods from a variety of others. The approach is primarily educational, focusing on helping the body heal itself naturally. The method uses natural processes, like sunlight, supplemented with diet and massage. The emphasis is on the whole person—physical, mental, emotional, social, and spiritual.

PERIMENOPAUSAL TREATMENTS

Many of the treatments previously described apply also to women who are perimenopausal. There are, however, important differences to consider as you progress through this life stage.

Medical Treatments

Most women who begin hormone replacement therapy do so when they begin to experience significant changes in their menstrual cycles. Their premenstrual symptoms may have increased in intensity, they may be having periodic hot flushes, they may be experiencing sleep disturbances, or they may be having sexual problems owing to either vaginal dryness or decreased desire. It is estimated that only about 15 percent of the women who need hormone replacement therapy are receiving it.

Preventing osteoporosis or coronary artery disease can motivate hormone replacement therapy. The usual practice, however, is to use hormone replacement therapy to alleviate perimenopausal difficulties. In general, estrogen replacement therapy can improve the following symptoms: vaginal dryness, urinary frequency and urgency, skin dryness, hot flushes, mood volatility, erratic memory, poor attention span, loss of sexual desire and responsiveness, migraines and other headaches, aches and pains, decrease in energy, sleep disturbances, heart palpitations, bone loss, hair thinning, and poor triglyceride ratios. Androgen replacement therapy (testosterone) can improve the following symptoms: decreased sexual desire and arousal, decreased mental clarity, decreased energy, hair thinning, and dysfunctional moods.

The combination of estrogen and androgens can, in general, augment some of the beneficial effects of estrogen alone. Estrogen replacement therapy has been found, however, to increase bone-mineral density and forestall osteoporosis in perimenopausal women. Natural progesterone (from wild yams) can improve the following perimenopausal symptoms: irregular bleeding, loss of bone density, and hot flushes. Progestins, however, have been found to have as many as thirty negative side effects. You must consult your physician in order to discover the right combination, delivery method, and dosages of these hormones.

If your uterus is still intact, you will probably begin with estrogen replacement, followed by progesterone replacement. Your physician may then recommend adding testosterone. Of course, each woman's needs are different, and the course of treatment must be personalized. If you have had a hysterectomy, you no longer are at risk for endometrial cancer, and estrogen, with or without testosterone, will make it unnecessary to replace progesterone. Replacing estrogen alone can lead to excessive uterine bleeding and intensified premenstrual symptoms. (See the section on medical treatments for PMS, above.)

Achieving the delicate balance between the ovarian hormones that your body is producing and those that you are receiving as therapy can be a difficult task. When these two sources do not complement each other effectively, some or all of your perimenopausal symptoms are likely to intensify. Psychological conflict, stress, changes in nutrition, and inappropriate exercise can exacerbate the imbalance. Achieving the balance you need may take some time. You need to be acutely aware of your peri-menopausal symptoms so that you can keep your physician informed about the effects of the hormone replacement therapy and so that you can evaluate our own self-treatments. The goal of treatment is not only symptom relief but also prevention of such conditions as heart disease, strokes, and osteoporosis. It can also help reduce the symptoms of dementia, such as those that charac-terize Alzheimer's disease.

There are several methods used for hormone replacement. The most common ones are oral preparations, transdermal patches, injections, vaginal creams, subcutaneous pellets, gels, vaginal estrogen rings, and intrauterine progesterone devices.

Oral preparations come in pill form and are ingested one or more times each day. Oral preparations have received the most research attention. One finding is that oral estrogen can improve the HDL/LDL ratio, a key indicator of cholesterol difficulties. They must pass through the intestines and liver, however, and if you have any problems in these functions, you may not receive the full benefits of the hormone replacement. The absorption rate may be uneven and unpredictable.

Transdermal patches stick on the skin (abdomen or buttocks) under your clothing. They may be changed as often as every three days or may last for a week. Transdermal patches are convenient, since they do not have to be changed very often. They release the hormone into circulation at a steady rate of absorption. The hor-mone does not pass through the gastrointestinal system or the liver, so women with liver or gastrointestinal problems can use this method. Some women develop skin irritations from these patches, and some have difficulty with transdermal absorption.

Injections are administered by a health-care professional into muscle tissue. A dose can last from one week up to three months.

Injections are used infrequently. This method is inconvenient since it requires the services of a health-care professional. An advantage of this approach is that the hormone is absorbed over a long period of time.

Vaginal creams are inserted with a syringe. Vaginal creams are easy to apply, and women use them usually three times per week or less. They are used primarily to treat vaginal difficulties, and the method does not provide the same level of protection for other perimenopausal symptoms as other methods do. Large doses can have negative side effects, and small ones often do not provide sufficient hormone replacement for cardiovascular protection and prevention of bone loss.

Subcutaneous pellets are inserted in fatty tissue under your skin by a health-care professional. These pellets may last for up to six months. Subcutaneous pellets require the services of a health-care professional, and this increases the cost as compared with oral preparations. The advantage is a slow, consistent release of the hormone for up to six months.

Gels are substances that you rub on your abdomen or thighs, usually once or twice each day. Gels (body creams) are convenient in that they are self-administered topically. You have to use more substance to get the required dosage. There is insufficient research on their effectiveness in treating perimenopausal symptoms.

Intrauterine progesterone devices are inserted into the endometrial lining of the uterus by a health-care professional. They release the hormone for six to twelve months. Intrauterine progesterone devices require the services of a health-care professional, adding to the cost of this method. This approach offers promise of treating endometrial hyperplasia or irregular bleeding without having the side effects of oral progesterone. The hormone is released over a long period of time, at a constant rate of absorption.

Hormone replacement therapy carries risks. There has been

much publicity surrounding its association with breast or endometrial cancer. However, research suggests that your chances of dying from coronary heart disease are ten times more (31 percent) than from breast cancer (about 3 percent), and your risk of dying from endometrial cancer is estimated at less than one percent. Since an early warning signal of endometrial cancer is heavy bleeding, you should seek medical advice if you are bothered by this symptom. Having high estrogen levels for a long time can lead to increased growth of the lining of the uterus, the endometrium, which can become malignant over time. The current preventive strategy is to combine estrogen with some form of progestogens (progesterone or progestins). This combination can assist in sloughing off the endometrium in a timely manner.

Women who are anticipating hormone replacement therapy may be afraid of breast cancer. The media has elicited this fear by drawing the public's attention to research that has been found to be flawed. The risk of breast cancer from HRT has not been definitively established. Although estrogen can stimulate increased growth of some existing tumors, the death rate from breast cancer is not higher for women who are taking estrogen supplements. Some research is pointing to progesterone as possibly contributing to the development of breast cancer. Other research suggests a genetic link to this type of cancer. Although the incidence of breast cancer increases after menopause, when estrogen levels decline significantly, it seems clear that replacing estrogen does not contribute to the risk. The regular use of mammography has reduced the mortality rate of breast cancer by about 30 percent.

The fear of contracting cancer as a result of HRT arose when dosages were much higher than they are today. Also, current practices emphasize combinations of hormones specifically calibrated to a woman's condition. Low dosages and new combinations of estrogen, progestins, and progesterone have reduced the risks significantly. Research and clinical practice is focusing not only on hormone levels but also nutrition, lifestyle, exercise, alcohol and tobacco intake, and environmental pollutants that can cause cancers. Research into genetics has focused on isolating information that can show predispositions to various types of cancer, and the results appear promising.

Deciding about hormone replacement therapy requires you to weigh your own symptoms and history and receive counseling that will help you consider the benefits and risks associated with the treatments. You are most likely to go through the treatment faithfully if you have confidence in your health-care practitioner, understand your needs, and learn about the benefits and potential risks involved.

Monitoring your regimen must include recording your treatments and blood chemistry. Here is a typical sequence of hormone replacement therapy:

1. You report changes in premenstrual or menstrual symptoms to your physician.
2. Your physician analyzes your ovarian (progesterone, testosterone, estradiol, LH, and FSH) and adrenal (DHEA-S) hormones through a blood panel.
3. You begin hormone replacement based on your reported symptom changes or abnormal hormone levels.
4. After a trial of hormone replacement, during which you monitor your symptoms, you get a second blood panel if you still report symptom difficulties.
5. Before making significant treatment changes, additional blood panels are usually helpful.
6. You undergo a continuous process of blood chemistry monitoring in order to maximize treatment effectiveness.

Numerous preparations are available for self-treatment, but they may not meet standards for approval by the Food and Drug Administration (FDA). Two classes of products that women use are natural progesterone (extract of wild yam) and phytoestrogens. Some women treat their PMS as well as perimenopausal symptoms by using the wild yam extract. Phytoestrogens, extracted from a variety of plants (soybeans, dong quai, and ginseng), may be helpful for mild symptoms, but they do not prevent osteoporosis or difficulties with cognitive functioning. It is virtually impossible to regulate your hormones by using these plant-based remedies. The dosages are difficult to ascertain, since the products do not come in standard, comparable forms. Also, you may not know how well you are achieving balance, and you may continue to have discomfort with perimenopausal symptoms in spite of your treatment. The term *natural* appeals to women who may be turned off by anything synthetic. What you need in hormone replacement therapy is to take in hormones that mirror those that your body produces whether or not they are labeled "natural" or "synthetic."

Oral contraceptives may ensure regularity in your menstrual cycle, in addition to preventing unplanned pregnancies and lowering the risk of ovarian cancer. Low dose oral contraceptives can have a cardiovascular benefit and produce greater bone mass and density. If, however, you smoke regularly, have diabetes or hypertension, or have other medical disorders, you may not be a candidate for the use of oral contraceptives.

Psychotherapeutic Treatments

The concerns that women express to therapists as they go through the perimenopausal years include the following:

- Aging
- Physical attractiveness
- Reevaluation of life purpose
- Changing relationships
- Career development
- Coping with perimenopausal symptoms
- Change in reproductive capacity
- Changing physical limitations

The most common treatments are individual, couples, and group sessions, and sometimes in combination. The length of treatment varies widely, depending on the initial problems and the patient's willingness and ability to follow through. Treatment often focuses on the kinds of concerns that women face during midlife, in conjunction with hormonal changes that they are experiencing. Psychotherapy explores the impact that these experiences are having on both intimate and other relationships. It is often important to involve others in the process, particularly significant others, in order to develop the support that women need through these physiological and psychological changes.

Group sessions are often organized for perimenopausal women and feature education as well as therapy. The educational sessions often are thematic; that is, each meeting includes information and discussion concerning a selected topic relevant to perimenopause, such as mood, cognition, sexual functioning, stress, and so on. Group therapy usually consists of working through the difficulties that members are facing in their daily lives, with consideration given to hormonal change.

Nutritional Treatments

All of the information discussed under PMS treatments above applies equally to perimenopausal women. Many women report that their perimenopausal changes benefit from the use of nutritional supplements. These supplements are not a substitute for hormone replacement, however, so consult your physician concerning their proper use. A number of foods and herbs contain phytoestrogens, which may reduce the impact of lowered ovarian estrogen production. Examples of these nutritional treatments include the following:

- Selected fruits (cherries, apples, coconuts, plums, and olives)
- Legumes (soybeans and peanuts)
- Soy products (tofu, miso, etc.)
- Almonds
- Tubers (carrots and yams)
- "Nightshade" foods (eggplant, tomatoes, potatoes, and peppers)
- Grains (cereals—especially wheat germ, but not rye, buckwheat, or white rice)
- Fennel, anise, and licorice

If you are perimenopausal, you should avoid the food substances listed under Table 13-1.

Food supplements become increasingly important as you age. Consult a nutritional specialist regarding your specific needs. Herbal treatments that you ingest can contain a number of traditional remedies that can be combined to control perimenopausal symptoms and to resolve imbalances in your body's organ systems,

SYMPTOM	HERBAL TREATMENT
Heavy bleeding	Vitex, flaxseed, lady's mantle, wild yam root, false unicorn root, and chaste tree
Hot flushes	Chickweed, dandelion, elderflower, licorice root, black cohosh root, wild yam root, chaste tree, false unicorn root, and motherwort
Sleep disturbances	Hops and chamomile
Cognitive dysfunction (memory, mental clarity, etc.)	Ginseng
Low energy	Ginseng, cinnamon, ginger, huang qi, dang qui, shatavarti, and sage
Mood swings	Motherwort and black cohosh
Low sex drive	Myrrh, peppermint, cayenne pepper, cloves, rosemary, ginger, garlic, cinnamon, and parsley
Dry skin	Comfrey, rose, and chamomile
Vaginal dryness	False unicorn root, black cohosh, hops, sage, calendula, and motherwort

Table 13-2

such as the ovaries and adrenal glands. See Table 13-2. Both food supplements and herbal treatments can be powerful agents, and you should take care in selecting them. Consulting clerks in food and vitamin stores can provide you a great deal of misinformation. You need to consult a nutritional specialist before beginning a program that includes these potions. Some "naturopath" professionals combine nutrition counseling, acupuncture, and advice on food supplements and herbs.

The herbs used to treat PMS, particularly vitex, black cohosh root, licorice root, chamomile, and motherwort, are also employed to alleviate perimenopausal symptoms. Some herbal treatments are targeted at specific perimenopausal symptoms.

Exercise Treatments

The amount of exercise that each woman needs does not change significantly as she ages. During perimenopause, however, there is the chance of weight gain, so exercise may be more important, since it increases your metabolism. Endurance exercise and weight training enhance bone mass and density. Women who exercise intensively, such as professional athletes, may stop having periods. Although they may develop high muscle endurance, their bone mass and density may suffer in the process, so exercise alone is not sufficient to protect the body from the long-term effects of the loss of ovarian and adrenal hormones. Exercise protects your cardiovascular system and improves glucose tolerance. Women report that exercise lessens the intensity of their perimenopausal symptoms. As in the case of women who have not entered the perimenopausal phase of their lives, exercise improves the sense of well-being, mood, and energy level.

Alternative Treatments

All the information discussed under "Treating PMS," above, applies equally to perimenopausal women.

WHAT YOU CAN DO ABOUT HYSTERECTOMY AND OOPHORECTOMY

In Chapter 10 we discussed the "ins and outs" of this surgical experience. Here are some things to consider if you decide to undergo this operation.

Prepare for the experience. Experiment by imagining not having a uterus. Then experiment by imagining not having ovaries. What images and anticipated changes arise in your mind? What are the losses and gains for you? Study information on the procedure so that you understand what you will be experiencing during and after the surgery. Discuss the surgery with your medical health-care providers, so that there are no surprises after the surgery and you feel a part of the team.

Set up a support system for yourself. Get others to help you prepare for the surgery and take care of you afterward. You will be making a number of adjustments during your recovery, and you may need others to be sensitive to and support you in going through this process.

Grow through the experience. Having a hysterectomy or oophorectomy can be a life-changing experience. You need to make sure that your view of yourself is positive and strengthening. Going through this experience is not necessarily traumatic. Some women have little or no difficulty with it, but others may find it stressful. Learn to think about pain as a healing force as well as a sign of danger. You may need to work with a psychotherapist to process this experience and turn it into useful learning for yourself.

Go beyond the experience. It is important to let go of having gone through a hysterectomy. You will adjust to not having periods and not birthing children. This can give you a strong sense of freedom.

What You Can Do About Your Moods and Cognitions

Chapters 3 and 4 discussed how your mood states and thinking can be affected by PMS and perimenopause. Here are some things that you can do to manage these symptoms:

Keep a record. This can assist you in answering the question, Are my moods and thinking patterns related to my menstrual cycle? Make notes when your medications or dosages change, and correlate them with your moods and cognitive symptoms. Also record other events, such as significant things that happen to you at work, your home life, your internal conflicts, and so on.

Tell others. Although it may be embarrassing at first, you may want to learn to share your menstrual cycle–related symptom profile with others whom you trust or whom you need to relate to closely.

Analyze your strategies. Reflect on what you do to help or hinder yourself as you cope with mood and cognition changes during PMS and perimenopause. You may decide to change some things that you do, discontinue others, or put more energy into others.

Try new approaches. Listen to your feelings in order to make decisions more fully. Pay attention to what your body is saying to you. You may discover this by noticing nonverbal cues in your behavior. For example, if you are leaning toward the door, you may want to leave. Ask yourself questions such as this, "If my tight shoulders could talk, what would they be saying right now?" Also pay attention to how rational you are being. You may be making excuses, distorting facts, blaming others, making unfounded assumptions, or otherwise thinking in a muddled manner. Introduce rationality into your decision making by debating the choices confronting you. Insist that each "side" base its argument on facts.

Ask for help. You may consult with your friends, family, physician, psychotherapist, physical trainer, or alternative health-care providers in order to develop a program for yourself. You may need a thorough physical examination, including an analysis of your blood chemistry. In addition, you may need to begin a program of medications to control your moods and cognitive functioning. You will need to make sure that your regimen is properly coordinated if you take an antidepressant or anti-anxiety agent in combination with hormone replacement and perhaps additional medications, food supplements, and herbal treatments.

MANAGING STRESS, BURNOUT, AND LIFE EVENTS

Handling stress effectively requires you to take charge of those situations that create stress for you. This means taking positive steps to strengthen your ability to manage difficult situations. Think of stress as coming both from your bodily functions and factors in your environment, such as other people, jobs, and so on. Both PMS and perimenopause generate marked changes in your mood, cognition, and behavior, and these changes can result in increased stress.

Monitor the subtle changes within yourself. This includes your ovarian-related cycles and emotional and cognitive fluctuations.

Observe your patterns of responding. Note carefully how you usually react, emotionally or behaviorally, when a general stressful event or a particular stressor occurs.

Learn how to increase your sensitivity to the factors that can lead to burnout. Develop a program to ensure that your self-concept remains positive, that you get rid of self-defeating habits, keep quality in your close relationships, and challenge the stress that often is present in work situations.

Move from inactive or reactive to proactive, or assertive. Taking charge of managing your stress and avoiding burnout requires that you take positive steps instead of waiting for situations to improve on their own. You may choose to attend an assertiveness training seminar to develop these skills.

Learn how to relax through breathing and visualization techniques. Tension is increased when we stop breathing or breathe shallowly in stressful situations. You can learn more relaxing responses through simply telling yourself to breathe deeply before reacting. You can also "rehearse" your responses to stress beforehand, developing a clear image of yourself performing effectively. You may also learn to bring into your consciousness an image of a safe place and let that image calm you while facing difficult situations.

Look into other sources of relief. Exercise often reduces stress. Confiding in your friends may "take the load off." Bubble baths, time alone, engaging in favorite activities, spending time in an intimate relationship, distracting yourself with work tasks, engaging in sports, watching television or movies—use your imagination.

Consider professional help. You may benefit from talking with a therapist if your responses to internal and external stressors exceed your capacity to cope effectively. You might also consider alternative treatments, such as massage, acupuncture, and acupressure.

Avoiding Burnout

Burnout depletes your energy. You function at levels below what is normal for you. Employing methods such as the following can help you prevent this serious personal condition. In *Managing Your Energy* (HRD Press, 1996), Jones & Bearley developed a list of practices that you can use to avoid this debilitating condition that we discussed in Chapter 6.

Focus on options. You do have options, and that is energizing. Focus on the choices available to you.

Set goals and make plans. This is axiomatic. We are much better at keeping ourselves energized if we know where we are going. Like the old bromide says, "If you don't know where you're going, any road will get you there."

Accept the givens. Moaning and groaning about the economy and about "what happens if the hills slide?" is de-energizing. Accept the fact that you work in a company where there is a lot of pressure and that you are working in an economy that is somewhat less than perfect.

Focus on a better world. Obviously the world is in pretty bad shape. However, the world that we live in is getting better—better transportation, better communication, better food, and better medicine. You can maintain your personal energy by focusing on what is improving.

Maintain optimism. A person with little hope does not maintain energy adequately.

Set yourself up to be successful. Take challenges that you are pretty certain you are going to be able to meet.

Live by this rule: "When in doubt, confront, when all else fails, try honesty." In other words, if you are having problems with somebody, go to him or her, look the person in the eye, and say, "Let's talk. We need to work this thing out."

Reward yourself. When you do something that is difficult for you, give yourself a reward. Other people may not notice, or they may not know how tough it is for you to do a particular thing. Instead of making yourself vulnerable by waiting for them to notice, reward yourself.

Value the importance of your work. Some people do not think that their work is important. If a person values making money or having a house at the lake, then the work itself does not nurture the person. Put your work into a larger context, and you will treat yourself better. Focus on the purpose of your work, how it contributes to others. Believe in what you are doing.

Focus on the "here and now." Don't look back at the "good old days." There is a good chance that those times were not as good as they are today. Concentrate on what is before you right now.

Turn off your motor every now and then. Learn how to waste time. "Type A" people often seem to be going ninety miles an hour all the time. Sometimes you need to rest, to relax, to reflect, and to re-energize yourself.

Confide in other people. All significant information about you should be known to some collection of others. That doesn't mean that you should get yourself a therapist. It does mean you have to "let it out" to avoid keeping secrets. If there is anything significant about you in relation to your significant other, go to the source.

Engage in self-analysis. Stop every now and then and ask, "Where am I going, what is going on here, who am I these days?"

Remind yourself that you are not the target. If you are a leader, some people will get angry with you. You will be a scapegoat for people's problems. You may represent a system that other people feel is wrong. You are not the target. People make themselves angry—you can't. They make sense out of what happens to them. You can only take responsibility for what you do.

Keep everything in perspective. Try to put what is bothering you right now into a "big picture." Sometimes worries become trivial when viewed in a larger context.

Claim your higher self. Each of us has a higher self, or an ideal self. Some people call it a soul or spirit. Claim that part of yourself, and center on it.

Love yourself unconditionally. We all have our faults. If we can look at ourselves optimistically and pump up our positive self-esteem, we can maintain our personal energy effectively. Being unconditional about yourself means prizing yourself without regard for (not in spite of) your "warts."

IMPROVING RELATIONSHIPS

Keeping communications clear with significant people in your environment is not a simple task, but it is a worthwhile one. It demands that you pay close attention to improving your listening skills and becoming an active listener. You need to check your understanding of what others say. Your self-expression should promote understanding on their part. If there is tension in these relationships, the process becomes more challenging.

Becoming assertive is not the same thing as *acting aggressively.* When you stand up for your rights while honoring those of others and when you require others to respect your rights as a human being, you are acting assertively. This is not an unfeminine posture. It is simply clear communication. You do not have to communicate indirectly, but you probably will not have the kind of relationships you want if you frequently engage in angry, confrontational communications.

Every relationship difficulty is not your fault. You do not need to *take everything personally* and accuse yourself of causing all tension around you. Learn to separate what you initiate and what other factors contribute.

Another trap to avoid is *jumping to conclusions.* You can make yourself jealous, for example, simply by gaining a snippet of information and making numerous assumptions from it. This can lead to unwarranted conflict. The trick is to catch yourself early before you draw indefensible conclusions.

You may need to test your assumptions, assuming that you become aware of them. *Blaming yourself* for everything that happens in your relationships is as self-defeating as *denying blame* for what you contribute to conflicts.

You may also find yourself engaging in *withdrawal* and *avoidance.* When relationships become uncomfortable, you may tend to move away from the person, your feelings, or thoughts because you assume that the discomfort may lead to some catastrophe, such as a breakup, angry encounter, or sadness.

Focusing on the "here and now" is an antidote to this tendency. If you *dwell on the past* or imagine what could happen in the future, you take energy away from dealing with your present reality in a responsible, clear way.

Finally, you may have a tendency to screen all interactions with your associates in terms of "what's in it for me?" This tendency to *dominate attention* can be taxing on your relationships with others who have to cope with you rather than interact freely with you. Overcoming these barriers to effective communications in your close relationships may require professional assistance, since you may have developed your communication style over a number of years.

Improving relationships almost always involves cleaning up communications. It also means earning trust and confidence through being reliable, trustworthy, flexible, and open to their influence.

WHAT YOU CAN DO ABOUT SEX AND INTIMACY

There is interdependence between intimate, committed relationships and sexual satisfaction. If you are unfulfilled sexually, the relationship may suffer, and if the relationship is unsatisfying, you may not be motivated to engage in sex freely. You need to get clear on what satisfies both you and the person with whom you have a relationship. For example, if you want cuddling, and the other person wants a "quickie," you may feel needy afterwards. If, on the other hand, your partner likes to do things sexually that make you uncomfortable, your desire and arousal may suffer. You may need to discuss your preferences regarding foreplay, sexual fantasies, sexual "turn-ons," orgasms, and "afterplay," and come to a common understanding of how to best express your relationship sexually.

You may consider increasing your private time with your partner, romancing each other, playing together, and touching each other intimately. Reflecting on good times together, you may want to repeat those activities that led to sexual desire and arousal in the past. Be creative in making space for private, pleasurable encounters.

If your premenstrual or perimenopausal symptoms cause difficulties in your sex life, talking about them with your partner may make them more manageable and may help to avoid uncomfortable, embarrassing situations. You may develop strategies to work with such symptoms as mood and cognitive changes, involving your partner in empathizing with and supporting you. Such sharing and problem solving can greatly enhance the intimacy in your relationships, and this can lead to greater satisfaction in your sex life. If problems persist beyond your ability to improve them, you might consult with a psychotherapist who specializes in sexual difficulties.

Whether you are dating, in a committed relationship, having sex with more than one partner, engaging in extramarital affairs, or experimenting with different forms of sexual practices, you need to be sensitive to age-related changes in your menstrual cycle and your changing PMS and perimenopausal symptoms. Relationships that are characterized by trust and sensitivity require open dialogue, sometimes on such uncomfortable subjects as what is happening to you physiologically. You can contribute significantly to your sexual satisfaction by focusing on clear communication and a willingness to adjust to the other person's needs while remaining true to yourself.

Figure 13-1 is a brief self-assessment of your present condition regarding your sexual life.

Figure 13-1 Sexual self-assessment

CONDITION	I'M DOING OKAY ON THIS	THIS IS NOT RELEVANT TO ME RIGHT NOW	I NEED TO IMPROVE ON THIS
I have a positive attitude toward sex.			
I am knowledgeable about sexual matters.			
I know what turns me on.			
I am aware of what turns my partner(s) on.			
I enjoy my sexual fantasies.			
I know ways to achieve orgasm.			
I know how to give my partner(s) satisfaction.			
I communicate freely with my partner(s) on sex.			
I enjoy variety in sexual activities.			
I have sex as frequently as I want.			
My sexual desire is about at the level I like.			
I become sufficiently aroused to enjoy sex.			
I am satisfied with my ability to achieve orgasm.			

Figure 13-1 Sexual self-assessment *continued*

CONDITION	I'M DOING OKAY ON THIS	THIS IS NOT RELEVANT TO ME RIGHT NOW	I NEED TO IMPROVE ON THIS
I feel comfortable in initiating sex.			
I am responsive to my partner(s) sexual overtures.			
I communicate freely during sex.			
Being sexual with my partner(s) is important to me.			
I can focus on the "here and now" during sex.			
For me sex is an important way to express love.			
I am able to focus on the sensations of sex rather than simply waiting for a climax.			
I feel sexually adequate.			
I am comfortable in showing my body to my sexual partner(s).			
I believe that I am sexually desirable.			
I communicate clearly to my partner(s) about my sexual needs and preferences.			
I have put my sexual history in the past.			

After you have completed the above assessment, study the pattern of your responses. Pay particular attention first to the things on which you rated yourself as "okay." Give yourself credit for establishing and maintaining these positive conditions. Then choose two or three items from the column labeled, "I need to improve on this." Make a plan for your development in these areas. You may want to seek further information on these conditions and talk with friends about how they remain positive in these areas. You may, of course, also work with your sexual partner on improving these conditions. You may choose to talk these over with your health-care team as well.

PUTTING IT ALL TOGETHER

Being female means going through developmental stages that include PMS and perimenopause. These require you to pay attention to both physical and psychological well-being as you age. As your ovaries age, your career develops, and your relationships change and mature, you will need to be proactive. Being assertive in managing your own health-care and mental health can give you a sense of pride. Making decisions regarding PMS and perimenopause needs to be based on solid information, so it is important to keep up with the growing research literature. The task may seem daunting, but the effort is worth it.

The first chapter discussed a general model of physical and mental health with nine interdependent elements to pay attention to as you face the changes through life's continuum. Maintaining your health, relationships, and career changes is a life-long commitment. Fortunately, a wide array of services are available to you along your journey. Medical practitioners are becoming more holistic, and alternative methods are emerging to offer choices in your self-management. Taking charge of your overall health in a proactive way means marshalling the resources of medicine, psychotherapy, nutrition, and exercise to fit your immediate and long-range requirements. No one keeps a record of your overall health for you. That is your opportunity. As you coordinate the work of your health-care team, consider their advice and information and take personal responsibility to do what is right for you. You can expect change as you age, and it is vitally important that you take charge of decision making as you experience it.

Give yourself permission to be less than perfect. So long as you take personal responsibility for being the woman that you can be, you cannot expect your program to produce positive results all the time. There will be setbacks and days when you are too tired to care, and others may fail to support you when you need their assistance. Keeping your eyes focused on your personal goals, however, can generate rich rewards for you. You can bet that your body, your relationships, and your career will change. Taking charge means doing whatever it takes to achieve your goals. Throughout the process it is important to love yourself—unconditionally. Affirm your basic goodness and determination. And commit to action that is based on awareness and credible information.

suggestions for
further Reading

Allgeier, E.R., and A.R. Allgeier. *Sexual Interactions* 3rd ed. Lexington, Mass.: D.C. Heath, 1991.

Barbach, L. *For Each Other: Sharing Sexual Intimacy.* New York: NAC Penguin, 1984.

Barch, J.F., and P.A. Barch. *Prescription for Nutritional Healing* 2nd ed. Garden City, N.Y.: Arenz Publishing Group, 1997.

Batson, M.C. *Composing a Life.* New York: Penguin Books, 1989.

Friedman, R.C., ed. *Behavior and the Menstrual Cycle.* New York: Marcel Dekker, 1982.

Blumstein, P., and P. Schwartz. *American Couples: Money/Work/Sex.* New York: William Morrow, 1983.

Borysenki, J. *A Woman's Book of Life: The Biology, Psychology, and Spirituality of the Feminine Life Cycle.* New York: Riverside Books. 1996.

Chopra, D. *Ageless Body, Timeless Mind: A Quantum Alternative to Growing Old.* New York: Harmony Books, 1993.

Cox, K., and Schwartz, J. *The Well-Informed Patient's Guide to Hysterectomy.* New York: Dell, 1996.

Crenshaw, T.L. *The Alchemy of Love and Lust.* New York: G.P. Putnam's Sons, 1996.

Cutler, W. *Hysterectomy Before and After: A Comprehensive Guide to Preventing, Preparing for, and Maximizing Health After Hysterectomy.* New York: Harper & Row, 1990.

Cutter, R. *When Opposites Attract: Right Brain/Left Brain Relationships and How to Make Them Work.* New York: The Penguin Group, 1994.

Dawood, M., M.D. Yusolb, J. McGuire, and L.M Demers. *Premenstrual Syndrome and Dysmenorrhea.* Baltimore: Urban and Schwarzan, 1985.

Downing, C. *Journey Through Menopause: A Personal Rite of Passage.* New York: Crossroad, 1987.

Faludi, S. *Backlash: The Undeclared War Against American Women.* New York: Crown, 1991.

Friday, N. *The Power of Beauty.* New York: Harper Collins, 1996.

Friedan, B. *The Fountain of Age.* New York: Simon and Schuster,1993

Golub, S., ed. *Lifting the Curse of Menstruation: A Feminist Appraisal of the Influence of Menstruation on Women's Lives.* New York: Haworth Press, 1985.

Greenwood, S. *Menopause Naturally: Preparing for the Second Half of Life.* Volcano, Calif.: Volcano Press,1989.

Halprin, S. *Look at My Ugly Face.* New York: Penguin Group, 1995.

Harrison, M. *Self-Help for Premenstrual Syndrome.* New York: Random House, 1982.

Helman, J.R., and, J. LoPiccolo. *Becoming Orgasmic: A Sexual and Personal Growth Program for Women.* New York: Prentice Hall, 1976.

Jacobowitz, R.S. *150 Most-Asked Questions About Middle Age, Sex, Love and Intimacy.* New York: Alfred A. Knopf, 1995.

Kanen, B. *Hormone Replacement Therapy, Yes or No?: How to Make an Informed Decision About Estrogen, Progesterone, and Other Strategies for Dealing with PMS, Menopause and Osteoporosis* 4th ed. Novato, Calif.: Nutrition Encounter, 1996.

Landau, C., M. Cyr, and A. Moulton. *The Complete Book of Menopause.* New York: Berkeley, 1994.

Lark, S. *Premenstrual Syndrome Self-Help Book.* Berkeley, Calif.: Celestial Arts, 1993.

Lee, J. R. *Natural Progesterone: The Multiple Roles of a Remarkable Hormone.* Sebastopol, Calif.: BLL Publishing.1993.

Levinson, D.J. *The Seasons of a Woman's Life.* New York: Alfred A. Knopf, 1996.

LoPiccolo, J., and L. LoPiccolo. *Handbook of Sex Therapy.* New York: Plenum, 1978.

Love, S. M., with K. Lindsey. *Dr. Susan Love's Hormone Book.* New York: Random House, 1997.

McIntyre, A. *The Complete Woman's Herbal: A Manual of Healing Herbs and Nutrition for Personal Well-Being and Family Care.* New York: Henry Holt, 1994.

Michael, R.T., Gagnon, J.H., Laumann, E.O., and Kolata, G. *Sex in America: A Definitive Survey.* New York: Warner Books, 1994.

Money, J., and A.A. Ehrhardt. *Man and Woman: Boy and Girl.* Baltimore: Johns Hopkins University Press, 1982.

Nachtigall, L.E., and J.R. Heilman. *Estrogen: The Facts That Can Change Your Life.* New York: Harper Collins, 1995.

Norris, R.B., and C. Sullivan. *PMS: Premenstrual Syndrome.* New York: Berkeley, 1983.

Ornstein, R., and D. Sobel. *The Healing Brain and Breakthrough Discovery About How the Brain Keeps Us Healing.* New York: Simon and Schuster, 1987.

Regalson, W., and C. Cotman. *The Sugar-Hormone Promise: Nature's Antidote to Aging.* New York: Simon and Schuster, 1976.

Reinisch, J.M., and Beasley, R. *The Kinsey Institute New Report on Sex: What You Should Know to Be Sexually Literate.* New York: St. Martin's Press, 1990.

Reinisch, J.M., L.A. Rosenblum, and S.A. Sanders. Eds. *Masculinity/ Femininity: Basic Perspectives.* New York: Oxford University Press, 1987.

Rossi, E.L. *The Psychology of Mind-Body Healing: New Concepts of Therapeutic Hypnosis.* New York: W. W. Norton, 1986.

Schiff, I. with A. B. Parson. *Menopause: The Most Comprehensive, Up-to-Date Information Available to Help You Understand This Stage of Life, Make the Right Treatment Choices, and Cope Effectively.* New York: Times Books, 1996.

Sheehy, G. *New Passages: Mapping Your Life Across Time.* New York: Ballantine, 1982.

———. *Pathfinders.* New York: Bantam Books. 1995.

———. *The Silent Passage.* New York: Random House. 1991.

Strausz, I.K. *You Don't Need a Hysterectomy: New and Effective Ways of Avoiding Major Surgery.* New York: Addison-Wesley, 1993.

Tannen, D. *You Just Don't Understand: Women and Men in Conversation.* New York: Ballantine, 1990.

Thoele, S.P. *Autumn of the Spring Chicken: Wit and Wisdom for Women in Midlife.* Berkeley, Calif.: Conari Press, 1993.

Utian, W.H., and R. Jacobowitz. *Managing Your Menopause.* New York: Simon and Schuster, 1990.

Vliet, E. *Screaming to Be Heard: Hormonal Connections Women Suspect . . . and Doctors Ignore.* New York: Evans, 1995.

index